Acknowledgements

We are grateful to Diane Simper and Elizabeth Walton for their help with the manuscript, whereas the faults belong solely to us; the book is that much better after their input. Our colleagues and students at Sheffield Hallam University and the University executive team have been instrumental in the development of Small Changes in recent years and we are grateful for the support. Finally the participants from our many programmes and the volunteers and paid staff who have worked as facilitators over the years, who have both shown such resolve in trying to tackle a problem that often has plagued clients for many years. These clients still have the fortitude to strive for change: even after many failed attempts. This book is dedicated to all our 'Small Changers'.

Small Changes (key behaviour change skills for weight management professionals)

Trevor Simper and Jean O'Keeffe with contribution from Helen Berry

Table of Contents

CHAPTER 1 INTRODUCTION

Learning Objectives to:

- Introduce the content of the book
- Understand why a 'behavioural' approach to weight-management is helpful
- Introduce the 'Small Changes' / Motivational Interviewing approach as an example of effective weight management

What's in this book?

This book covers skills and practices for successful weight-management practice. It synthesises evidence from the scientific literature base i.e. research articles in peer-reviewed publications with our own experience of running a weight-management service, conducting research and training others in weight-management over many years. Each chapter begins with learning objectives and ends with an assessment, designed to check these learning objectives. Chapters 1-8 also contain real life case-studies taken from the authors' weight-management practice.

For whom is this book Intended?

In effect this book is the manual for a behavioural change approach to weight-management and a book for:

- students in universities studying exercise, nutrition and lifestyle related subjects
- a manual for counsellors in the NHS and private practice

- a resource for lecturers

The scope of our weight problem: the obesity agenda

In January of 2010 a cross-government strategy costing £372 million was launched to tackle obesity. 'Healthy Weight, Health Lives' is designed to bring together employers, individuals and communities to promote healthy eating, physical activity and health at work. It aims to halt the accelerating rates of obesity seen UK-wide, and commits to help provide effective treatment for and support of individuals who are overweight or obese.

With 66% (and rising) of our population overweight or obese, it is now 'normal' to be overweight- and judging by the proliferation of products, TV programmes and books on the subject, weight is clearly important to many of us. Obesity is widespread in the western world. The number of people in the United Kingdom, who are either overweight or obese, according to the Body Mass Index, means that it is now 'normal' to be overweight in the UK (DOH, 2010). Health problems connected with being overweight are numerous with cardiovascular disease, type II diabetes and certain types of cancer being most prominent. The focus of interventions suggested by the Foresight report (Foresight group 2007) should be on prevention of weight gain in children, changes to food policy, changes to the built environment and weight-management with the intention of preventing illness and disease for those already overweight.

Yet the prevalence of overweight and obesity in the western world calls for treatment and prevention of worse health in those already overweight/obese as well as addressing issues with the built environment, policies and strategies for public transport, sport, physical activity, food production, marketing and many aspects of society from school dinners to familial modelling (Foresight, 2007).

Weight management programmes for those already overweight or obese are numerous, interventions range in length from a few weeks to, more rarely, programmes lasting over a year. A commonality amongst the results from studies of such interventions is a high rate of recidivism (dropout). The length of treatment may be very important in the long-term success of an intervention, with a year or so of intervention yielding better results than short-term interventions and 2 years of intervention failing to produce further results (Peri *et al.*, 1989, 1997). Some interventions use physical activity promotion alone, some use nutritional education alone and some both together. Interventions may also combine physical activity and/or nutrition with behaviour change techniques. The relative effectiveness of each combination has been scrutinised, and it may well be that using nutrition, exercise and a behavioural approach in combination holds the key to the most successful ingredients for a weight-management programme (Soderlund et al 2009; Peri et al 1984, 1997).

Definition of success is key in establishing whether a programme is 'successful' or not (Wing & Hill 2001). The high rates of recidivism may cause pessimism amongst those seeking to manage weight; however, achievable weight loss of 5-10% of starting bodyweight has important clinical benefit and has long been shown to be a more sustainable achievable goal than dramatic weight loss (Egger 1997).

The National Institute for Health and Clinical Excellence (NICE) provide guidelines for health professionals and community based interventions that seek to tackle weight-management and behaviour change (NICE, 2006, NICE, 2007). These documents provide essential guidance for weight-management programmes carried out in the community as they give clear clinical rationale for procedures necessary to ensure a sustainable project aimed at improving lifestyle. Programmes could and indeed should observe these areas of guidance in order to assist in developing and delivering robust interventions. Key advice includes:

Overview of the Governmental Reaction To Obesity

The acknowledgment of obesity, as a major health risk, was in response to the high incidence of heart disease, diabetes and other lifestyle diseases in the Western world.

Projected statistics show that by 2050 we can expect the percentage of obese men between the ages of 21 – 61, to reach 90% from the 2007 level of 70%. In 2007 30% of women between the ages of 21 – 61 were obese. The projected figure for adult women in 2050, is 80%.

The percentage of obese boys between the ages of 6 – 10 in 2007 was 25%. This is expected to rise to 60% in 2050. Of girls between the same ages in 2007, 22% were obese. In 2050 this figure may be 55% (Jebb 2011).In short there seems little doubt that we have increased dramatically in bodyweight in recent decades and continue to do so.

Initial Governmental Reaction

Part of the initial response to obesity was a straightforward idea to tell people what was wrong and how to put it right. The bald, `Eat Less, Move More', order has been prolifically distributed with instructions. More apparently simple suggestions included the eating of fruit and vegetables. 'Five a Day' is one of the key national healthy-eating campaigns. Many people are not eating a variety of fruit and vegetables and are also stumped on how big was a portion. Many actively dislike fruits and potatoes are the only vegetable recognised as worth putting on the table.

Five portions a day, (which includes a glass of fruit juice, frozen, dried and tinned produce) was settled on as the number most likely to be accepted as a possible, reachable target. The suggestion of 5-9 nine portions is less well known, as five a day seems is a tall order amongst a population eating only 2-3 portions a day.

The attempt to bring the healthy message, to every inhabitant in the United Kingdom, did succeed in capturing the attention of more of the population; a population that overall still does not eat sufficient fresh or frozen fruits and vegetables.

It is difficult to imagine that any previous generation paid more attention to the amount, quality and effects of what we eat. Food, its preparation and consumption, is one of the most frequent topics of our conversations. Children are arriving home from school offering healthy choice guidelines to their parents. 'Teacher says a banana is better for me than crisps!' Cook and eat campaigns have lured more men into the kitchen as day to day food preparation and presentation skills gain a higher status. The TV schedule is populated with cooking programmes and still we get fatter.

Foresight, the Government Office for Science identifies several factors strongly related to the development of obesity:

Transport
Education
Parental control
Stress
Convenience
Grazing
Habit
Food production
(Foresight group 2007).
All of these factors impact both at a national and individual level.

These factors are considered in the government and health authority's strategies to deal with rising obesity levels. Changes in transport, education and food production effect the population as a whole.

The body mass index (BMI) is used to calculate how overweight people are. BMI is weight in kilograms (kg) divided by height in metres squared (m^2). The World Health Organisation have outlined different categories of BMI with 25-29.9Kgm^2 equalling overweight, 30-39.9 Kgm^2 signalling obesity and >40 Kgm^2 representing morbid obesity.

Recommendations for physical activity and food differ internationally but are fairly similar (e.g. Australia and the

United States) to those in the United Kingdom. For those people who are or have been overweight or obese the recommendation is 60 minutes a day of moderate intensity activity on most days of the week. However the Health Survey for England in 2008 reports firstly very low levels of physical activity as per previous studies and uses accelerometry [1] to assess activity levels rather than self-report. The results based on measures for representative samples suggest that self-reports are probably over-reported. The accelerometry data suggests that only 6% of men and 4% of women met the government's guidelines for physical activity.

Recommendations also exist for strength training (one set of 10-15 repetitions of between 8 and 10 exercises performed 2-3 days a week). Resistance exercise augments the benefits gained from aerobic training in that it is protective to lean tissue, bone mineral density and results in higher metabolic rates as a result of the additional lean tissue (Surgeon General 1996) and improvements to blood sugar control Mcrdle Katch and Katch (2007). Within the data for physical inactivity there appears no information on how many people engage with exercise that is protective in relation to lean tissue, bone health and balance in the elderly. As our occupations have become less physically demanding and lifting, carrying and strength type activity has reduced

---

[1] An accelerometer is a monitor which counts energy expenditure when attached to the user, like a pedometer but more sophisticated measuring cycling running walking an energy output not just steps

(both in the home and at work) strength training has become more of an issue- sarcopenia (loss of muscle tissue) is of particular concern in the elderly and infirm.

Accurate dietary analysis is notoriously difficult to achieve, however, most people in the UK population probably do not eat the minimum recommended level of at least five portions (400g) of fruit and vegetables recommended by the World Health Organisation (Nishida *et al.*, 2004).

Overweight is ultimately a result of energy intake exceeding energy needs. Genetic differences do occur between individuals but these are seemingly only now expressed as societal changes to energy use and consumption have come about.

Often the weight loss methods employed by individuals are sizeable departures from 'normal' life; life the way we usually live it, based on our up-bringing, beliefs, culture, relationships, tastes, income and where we live. Consider the people you know. Is there anyone who is exactly like you? Is there anyone who has; the same way of doing things, reacts to everything the way you do, enjoys the same food, has the same abilities and strengths as you? This is how we settled on 'small' changes i.e. a 5-10% alteration to diet and physical activity uptake is manageable but a 30-50% change may not be.

Apart from identical twins, who may share everything from appearance to thoughts, most of us are so varied we would be hard pressed to recognise who belongs to which family.

While there is evidence relating physiology and genetic inheritance (Bouchard et al. 1990) to rates of weight gain (i.e. the rates of weight loss/gain are the same between monozygotic*[2] twins but *not* the same between unrelated adults) we clearly gain and lose weight at different rates even when we eat the same amount of food and do the same amount of exercise as another person. Attitudes and habits around food and activity are also almost certainly influenced by our surroundings - little people who grow up with overweight parents are very likely to become overweight in the same way that children of smokers are more likely to become smokers. People who live with overweight people will more likely become overweight themselves (and vice versa when living with thin people). The grades of University students are affected more by the people they share a room with, more than they are by the number of points the student has when they arrive at University! (Thaler and Sunstein 2008).

This leads us onto an important element of Small Changes which is to '*work within the context of the client's life*' Therefore it is about you being a bit fitter, leaner healthier irrespective of the genetic hand you've been dealt.

---

[2] Monozygotic twins are identical i.e. one zygote splits and forms two embryos

But People *Do* Lose Weight

The good news is, we *do* know how people have lost weight and maintain that loss. These 'secrets' to use an advertising term have been discovered by asking individual people how they succeeded. Although the range of differences between people is wide, there are common denominators that apply to them all – the 'most people' principle. Naturally the range of achievement is also wide as it partly depends on the individual starting point and on personal goals.

The National Weight Control Registry (NWCR) based in the United States is the clearest example of a project to explain how successful weight managers have achieved and maintained weight loss, the registry has a membership of more than 5000 people, 80% of whom are women and 20% men. The members have lost an average of 66 lbs. (4st 10lb) and kept it off for five and a half years.

These are averages (within which there is a lot of diversity) Weight losses have ranged from 30lbs (2st 2lb) to 300 lbs. (21st 6lb). The duration of maintaining this weight loss has ranged from 1 to 66 years.

The NWCR has analysed how the weight loss was accomplished:

- o 45% of registry participants lost the weight on their own
- o 55% lost weight with the help of some type of programme
- o Some people have lost the weight rapidly

- Others have lost weight very slowly over as many as 14 years
- 98% of registry participants modified their food intake in some way
- 94% increased their physical activity, with the most frequently reported form of activity being walking
- Many eat breakfast every day (78%)
- Many check their weight regularly (at least once a week) to keep a check on progress (75%)
- Many watch less than 10 hours of TV per week (62%)
- The majority exercise, on average, for about 1 hour per day (90%)
- Most follow a diet lower in fat and do higher levels of activity than previously.
- When people take 'days off' (from exercising and eating well) this does not extend beyond two days

Different Weight-management Approaches

Weight loss in terms of behaviour is simple:

'Eat less, move more.'

This persistent and enigmatic mantra for losing weight may also leave people feeling unclear;

Eat?

Eat what? Eat when? How much? How often?

Move?

*How much should I move? When should I move? How often
should I move?*

Let's give ourselves a break here. Changes to the amount of
energy we expend and the way we eat are fairly recent. Just
a few decades have seen life change so much that we seem
suddenly fat. Perhaps we are now trying to re-dress the
balance. Essentially this means adapting and changing to
suit the new environment, so far we have done this by
getting fatter and seeing the increased prevalence of lifestyle
diseases. People may also wonder what the fuss is about. If
they have 'managed' their own weight and therefore have no
issue, they may also feel they have the answer for everyone
else! Live like me and you'll be ok! In effect this propagates
the potential for looking down on those fat and lazy people
who are overweight…We will attempt to unpack this
throughout the book and of course the answer is yes, we can
lose weight by eating less and moving more.   What we are
really emphasising is that whatever the technique a
individual uses it needs to be chosen by that person and not
by us.

Popular Techniques for Losing Weight

Taking fortified fluids, using the system of green days/free
days, buying products from private weight loss companies,
joining a gym, skipping, kettle-bells and removing
carbohydrates or fat entirely from the diet are all talked
about, written about and employed by people attempting
weight-management.

Small Changes - *An Example* of a Behavioural Approach

Small Changes participants only make changes that fit into the context of *their* lifestyle. Every change is chosen by the individual according to what they feel is the most important issue for them. A sensible approach, we suggest, will be designed to include every aspect of a participant's life, because every part of our lives interrelates and effects the whole. In short, real life is not consistently regular or organised. Unexpected events occur, accidents happen, schedules change and routines are disrupted.

By choosing the Small Changes that are feasible for them, the individual remains in control of their health decisions and will experience continuous success. A disruption is just that, something to deal with, to negotiate around, to accept until it passes.

Small Changes are easy to make and immediately effective both physically and mentally. Imagine the preposterous notion of blundering on with the insistence that workouts and attendance at the gym are 'best' for weight loss, this I likely to have a nullify-ing effect on the client who hates the gym/is disengaged with the idea of that type of exercise. A client who is facilitated will, perhaps, walk more and eat breakfast more often i.e. adopt behaviours which *they* control and choose for themselves, which result in long term weight behaviour change for that individual.

How does 'Small Changes' work?

Small Changes uses well-known counselling skills to facilitate clients in making their own decision around changes for weight-management. The Approach combines the expertise of behaviour change, nutrition and exercise. This way when client asks for advice we have people on hand to provide it, Small Changes has grown from our work, i.e. the of an experienced counsellor, Jean O'Keeffe and the work of a nutritionist/exercise scientist Trevor Simper, we have trained over the years in many approaches to psychological helping. In recent years we have adopted motivational interviewing as our preferred approach. There are good reasons for this: MI is an accessible approach that positively encourages people interested in applying behaviour change skills to their work. MI has nothing in its approach that contradicts what we have practised at Small Changes for years. MI also has a developing 'evidence base' for treating behaviours including success in weight-management (Armstrong, 2011).

Jean combined her skills with NHS Public Health Nutritionist Trevor Simper and around 2001 they began working together with other colleagues on what eventually became Small Changes. Later on Small Changes developed into a research project at Sheffield Hallam University. Various publications and projects have been run with many groups of individuals, (Simper, O'Keeffe, *et al.* 2008, 2009, 2010).

Our facilitators train via MI workshops when they have an existing nutrition and exercise degree or similar set of qualifications. This is an important base for anybody working in weight-management or running a weight management programme. We leave you to make up your own mind but propose a reasonable starting point for a weight-management professional is as follows:

- Nutrition and exercise related degree *(Or Experience and qualifications in this area that equate to having said degree)*

- Completion of behaviour change workshops *(for example, in our case we use beginning, intermediate and advanced MI workshops)*

- a one to two year period of supervised practice with an experienced supervisor *(where constant feedback from recorded sessions and observations are offered and reflective practice is carried out)*

We hasten to add here that MI is not the only approach that may be useful for weight management. Solution Focused Therapy or CBT may work well or a combination of approaches. We propose MI as a workable and effective approach suitable for lifestyle issues. MI was first proposed by Miller and Rollnick (1983) and offers an approach that deals with ambivalence and 'resistance' via a 'directive' client-centred counselling approach.

Case Study 1: Exploring Importance and Confidence

SC: *'Hi Joan thanks for coming to meet me today, I know you responded to the advert for people who were struggling to manage their weight could we start with you explaining a little about what's going on with your weight? '*

Joan: *'Ok, I started to gain weight five years again after the birth of my first child, it's gone up steadily* *since then and I'm now four stone heavier than I was before the kids'.*

SC: *'Your life changed a fair bit after having the children'.*

Joan: *'Yes, big time! I didn't have time for exercise I stopped eating the way I used to and basically my life revolved around getting the older one to and from nursery and looking after the baby at the same time and let me tell you that's tougher than working full time!'*

SC: *'People perhaps don't realise that, just how much work someone looking after two small children has to do'.*

Joan: *'No they don't. I think a lot of people think its easy being off work and just dropping kids off with child-minders etc and that was not it for me'.*

SC: *'Joan, now that you've gained the weight - how important on a scale on 1 to 10 would you say it is to start tackling this - with 1 being not important at all and 10 being very, very important? '*

Joan: *'10'*

SC: *'OK it's that important, you really want to do something about this'*

Joan: *'It's the most important thing right now, I feel awful I can't go clothes shopping, I feel bad to go out in public, you know like a slob? As if everyone's looking at me a saying look at that fat cow. I want to get back to where I was I am not this person. I am slimmer. It feels unfair to be working this hard looking after my kids and now working part-time as well and getting fatter at the same time.'*

SC: *'it seems like a contradiction, you're doing everything to care for your children and going to work and then gaining weight for your troubles, it seems unfair'.*

Joan: *'Exactly'*

Sc: *'Joan could you also tell me, using the same scale, how confident you are that you can change your lifestyle and effect your weight with 1 being not at all and 10 I definitely can'.*

Joan: *'Maybe I am a five'*

SC: *'OK a five why not a zero? How come you up at the half-way point?'*

Joan: *'Well I'm here to start this now and I know if I can just start to concentrate on my diet and activity I will be able to lose at least some of the weight'.*

Sc: '*I'm sure you're right. Maybe we should start to talk about how you want to go about this - what seems like the priority for you?*'

Chapter 1 Assessment (answers in appendix 1)

1. Only Motivational Interviewing can be used as a behavioural approach to weight-management T or F?
2. Small Changes prescribe the elements a client needs to change to most positively effect their weight T or F?
3. Small Changes is about facilitating the client in making her or his own decisions T or F
4. Small Changes seeks a 'guiding' approach i.e. we don't prescribe at all T or F
5. Advice is offered when it asked for or after we have obtained permission from the client T or F
6. 'Scaling' questions are an MI tool and help us to advise the client what to do? T or F?
7. Scaling questions help the client open up about an issue so that we might understand more clearly how motivated they are to change and how confident they are about making changes T or F?
8. Exploring motivation and confidence allows us opportunity to focus on positive aspects for moving forward
9. Advice is never needed in weight-management counselling T or F?
10. We all gain weight at the same rate and need the same interventions for weight loss in truth one size really does fit all T or F?

References

BOUCHARD C (1990) The Response to Long-term Overfeeding in Identical Twins *N Engl J Med*, **322**:1477-1482

DEPARTMENT of Health (2008), Healthy Weight Healthy Lives: a cross government strategy for England, last accessed October 2013

http://www.dh.gov.uk/en/Publicationsandstatistics/Publications/Publicati onsPolicyAndGuidance/DH_082378

EGGER, G. Swinburn B (1997) An 'ecological' approach to the obesity pandemic *BMJ* 315:477-480

MILLER, W.R and Rollnick, S (2002) Motivational interviewing, Preparing People for Change, Guildford Press.

National Weight Control Registry http://www.nwcr.ws/

NATIONAL INSTITUTE for HEALTH and CLINICAL EXCELLENCE (2006) Obesity: the prevention, identification, assessment and management of overweight and obesity in adults and children http://guidance.nice.org.uk/CG43

NATIONAL Institute for Health and Clinical Excellence (2007) Behaviour change at population, community and individual levels http://guidance.nice.org.uk/PH6/Guidance/pdf/English

NISHIDA et al. (2004) The Joint WHO/FAO Expert Consultation on diet, nutrition and the prevention of chronic diseases: process, product and policy implications. *Public Health Nutrition*: **7**(1A), 245–250

PAXMAN, J.R, Hall,A.C. Harden,C.J, O'keeffe, J, Simper, T.N (2011)Weight loss is coupled with improvements to affective state in obese participants engaged in behavior change therapy based on incremental, self-selected 'Small Changes' Nutrition Research

PERRI ,M.G. et al. (1984) Effect of a multicomponent maintenance program on long-term weight loss *Journal of Consulting and Clinical Psychology* 52, 3, 480-481

PERRI M G. Et al. (1989) Effect of length of treatment on weight loss. *Journal of Consulting and Clinical Psychology*, **57** (3), 450-452.

PRENTICE A.M, Jebb S.A (1995) Obesity in Britain gluttony or sloth? BMJ 311:437

SIMPER, T[1]. O'Keeffe, J[1,2]. (2009) Reduced energy intake and maintained loss of weight is observed at 6 months follow up of the **'Small Changes** Programme' *European Journal of Obesity* May Vol2,S2 p228

SIMPER, T[1], Paxman[1], J. O'Keeffe, J[2] (2008) Small-group weight-management programme using self selected goals improves General Well Being scores. *International Journal of Obesity*, May S2

SODERLUND. A, Fischer. A, Johannson, T (2009) Physical activity, diet and behaviour modification in the treatment of overweight and obese adults: a systematic review Perspectives in Public Health **129**(3)132-142

SURGEON General report (1996) Physical Activity and Health: A Report of the Surgeon General, Centers for Disease Control and Prevention, Atlanta

THALER, R.H, and Sunstein, C.R (2008) *Nudge Improving Decision About Health, Wealth and Happiness* Yale University Press New Haven

VANDENBROECK, P, Goossens, J., Clemens, M. (2007). Tackling Obesity- Future Choices – Building the Obesity System Map. London : Foresight, Government Office, London.

WING, R.R,HILL J.O (2001) Successful Weight Loss Maintenance *Annual Review of Nutrition* **21**: 323-341

CHAPTER 2

What should be included in a comprehensive weight-management programme?

Chapter Objectives to:

- Propose what should be included in comprehensive programmes

- Find ideas for structuring your own programme

- Clarify factors other than just 'weight lost' as important changes

- Gain an understanding of what is included in comprehensive programmes

In this chapter we offer a review of weight-management studies, in an attempt to answer the question 'How successful are weight-management programmes?' It is arguably important to include support for both ends of the energy equation, i.e. physical activity and food. It is also important to offer a clear behavioural change approach in a comprehensive programme. By clear we mean something that is traceable/repeatable by other deliverers. In the case of

Small Changes we explain in detail throughout this book what is done. Broadly a Rogerian counselling approach where clients are listened to and empathy is employed - clients are facilitated in making changes to their lifestyle. More recently we have adopted motivational interviewing as the method for treating clients. This allows our work in future to be replicated and understood by others as they can clearly see what is being done rather than describing it simply as 'behaviour change'. Approaches are quite rightly criticised for being a) unclear over what the actual behavioural approach is and b) when this is stated not having some way of checking 'treatment fidelity' which verifies that the approach is being adhered to (Breckon, 2004).

The 3 key factors for weight management

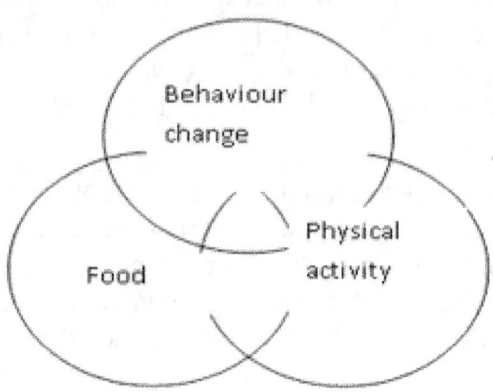

We argue that successful weight-management programmes will include measures of body-composition, weight, physical activity, nutrition *and* a relatively long period of follow-up. These factors can be said to be the constituents of a 'comprehensive' programme. 'Success' can be defined by positive changes in the above areas.

Background

Soderlund and Fischer (2009) scrutinised physical activity with/without diet and behaviour modification and found that a combination of exercise, diet and a 'behaviourial' approach is favourable. Sharma (2007) reviewed behavioural interventions in treating obesity in adults, recommendations based upon this review include that physical activity and nutrition behaviours must be approached together. This chapter also highlights the need for clear behavioural approach to underpin interventions. The difficulty where the theory is not clear relates to replicating the programme, identifying what has/has not worked. Based upon the results from this review Sharma also highlights the need for a treatment period of at least 6 months. We extend this by suggesting that 1 year is the minimum length to show more than short term change, importantly as nearly all weight lost in interventions occurs during the first six months, one year interventions also monitor 'maintenance'.

Success also needs qualification, with some rationale for a 'clinically significant' weight loss maintained for a certain period representing a reasonable indication of success e.g. 5-10% weight loss maintained for at least 1 year (Wing & Hill 2001). Some programmes consider body-composition and others do not. The review we present in this chapter attempts to evaluate the success (using agreed criteria to define success) of programmes which consider: body-composition, weight loss, sufficient length of treatment, inclusion of both physical activity and nutrition combined with a behavioural change approach.

Applying a psychotherapeutic approach to weight-management

There are different approaches to helping people in the sense of counselling. Often they have central themes like: asking open ended questions, really trying to listen to the client and gain their story, understanding the problem/s they face, using reflection and summaries, of what the client has said (to check the helper has heard correctly what the client means).

Here we pick an evidence based approach (MI) and both describe it, and then analyse what the scientific literature says about MI specifically in relation to weight-management.

Behaviour change training is something that professionals can begin to undertake at a basic level with a couple of days, or even a day-long seminar. It is worth noting though that really developing skills and competency in this area needs intense and long-term supervision. Hopefully this won't put you off getting started! MI for example can be started by attending a two-day workshop and you will feel like you are winning right from the start. That being said, becoming a skilled behavioural change counsellor is likely to take a couple of years of practising and being supervised practising and continuously reflecting on what you do to modify and develop practice.

Professionals reading this book are likely to have carried out a professional study/training of some type: medicine, nursing, health care, health promotion, fitness instruction, nutrition, lifestyle related studies etc. It is you, and I, that need effective behaviour change skills. Behaviour change skills augment our existing skills and knowledge around health, because ultimately these areas of professional practice are predicated upon us helping clients to *change* behaviour. A good effective behavioural change training is only going to help your professional practice and from my own personal experience (Trevor) in a major way! The one we are proposing here is Motivational Interviewing, it is in no way the only behaviour change approach but there is simply nothing within MI that we disagree with!

What is MI?

First proposed by Miller and Rollnick in 1982 (first published Miller 1983), MI is a 'client centred' approach to helping people change. The power of decision making rests with the client *not* the facilitator. MI is useful in helping clients establish their own motivation for change - this is the motivation in MI rather than you and I providing the motivation!

MI seeks to clarify the client's confidence to change as well as the importance of changing the target behaviour. Furthermore clients very often are 'ambivalent' in relation to behaviour, shown in this quote form one of our participants:

'I'd like to lose weight and feel fitter but I find exercise hard work and enjoy eating cheese cake on the sofa'.

Ambivalence is the see-saw part (i.e. people often feel two ways - or more than two ways - about maintaining or changing a situation/ behaviour). An MI counsellor might choose to reflect to the client with cheese cake/sofa problem the fact that although the client sees change as difficult, they clearly recognise and value feeling fitter and losing weight, this might encourage the client to talk more and clarify further just what would be so good about losing that weight and gaining fitness (rather than focussing on the attraction of the sofa and cheesecake!).

What does the evidence show around using MI for weight management?

Motivational interviewing offers promising results for maintenance of healthful behaviours and in recent years has been applied to weight loss and weight-management. It is fairly clear from the promising results so far that MI offers great potential for weight-management (Rubak, 2005; Armstrong, 2011: Van Dorsten, 2011). Rubak and colleagues conducted a meta-analysis (collating the results from different research trials and adding them together to see what the overall effect seems to be) and they concluded that in 75% of trials there were equal physiological and psychological effects and that participants from the trials using MI showed significant improvements to BMI, cholesterol, systolic blood pressure and blood alcohol but no significant results for cigarette smoking and HBA1C (a measure of the subjects blood sugar control). More recently Armstrong et al. 2011 conducted a review of MI for weight-management suggesting greater efficacy using MI over and above other approaches.

Weight loss success, resulting from MI treatment is, at least, as effective as results from 'other' behavioural weight loss approaches. Only one study suggests significantly more weight loss in an MI group and another suggests better glucose control when adding 3 MI sessions to a group of diabetic women receiving (Carels et al. 2007: Mhurchu et al. 1998 and Smith et al. 2007).

Body-composition and Proposal of a 'Quotient' Of Positive Change

It is, perhaps, reasonable to factor in body-composition using the judgement that fat loss equals positive weight change and lean loss equals negative change (therefore lean gain is considered positive). For example a subject loses 4 kilos, one of which is lean; their rate of positive 'change' would be 3 kilograms i.e. 4 kilograms -1 kilogram. If, in this scenario, the subject had lost 4 kilograms but also gained 1 kilogram of lean tissue then the lean increase plus fat loss would mean a positive 'change' of 5 kilograms had occurred. Lean tissue loss might be considered negative in weight loss programmes and especially where sarcopenia (loss of muscle tissue) and bone mineral density are key issues (Roubenoff 1997, Fried 2001) e.g. for post-menopausal women and the elderly who are at greater risk of osteoporosis. Physical activity has been shown to be protective of lean body tissue in older people, whether they lose weight or not, whereas weight loss without physical activity results in loss of 'functional' lean tissue Jansen et al. (2002).

Determining a quotient of change, i.e. what represents good, bad or excellent, will require an analysis of a large data set and needs a slightly more complex equation. For this purpose we propose a simple 'quotient of positive weight change', which is as follows: Lean change minus fat change minus .5% of the body-fat change equals the quotient of positive change i.e.: Lc-Fc - 0.5-% BFC = 'quotient of positive change'.

Physical Activity: fitness versus fatness

An increase in physical activity has been suggested to effect psychological well-being improvements (Fox, 1999) to the point of concluding that clinical depression can be effectively treated with exercise. Enhanced dietary intake proffers protection from disease *irrespective* of weight loss and the concept of 'health at any size' needs further exploration (Bacon et al. 2005). Seminal work has shown reduced risk of cardiovascular disease and correlated conditions in persons who, for instance, are physically active yet overweight (Paffenbarger, 1986).

Nutrition

Attention to nutrition for weight-management is paramount; the relationship between our eating habits and obesity however, is still unclear. Suggestions that the massive rise in people being either overweight or obese is due to gluttony are confounded by the suggestion that our calorie intake over decades has changed little or not at all and has maybe even declined (Prentice & Jebb, 1995). Despite this an energy imbalance is implicated in overweight and obese individuals. Genetic factors may explain individual differences in rates of weight gain amongst people following the same lifestyle i.e. levels of exercise and Kcal intake, (Bouchard, 1990) but the principal factors in the aetiology of overweight and obesity are considered to be environmental/behavioural rather than biological (Foresight group, 2007).

This leads to the conclusion that just concentrating on one part of the energy balance is nonsensical. Even if health gain and not weight loss is the target, nutrition impacts heavily on our risk of disease irrespective of weight. An example is given by Bazzano et al. (2008) who studied a large cohort of people and found that intake of green leafy vegetables and whole-fruit was inversely associated with type II diabetes development irrespective of BMI.

Treatment Length and Follow-up/ maintenance

Perri and colleagues (1989) first identified the effects of different lengths of treatment, in the 1980's, i.e. showing that there is an effect relating directly to the length of treatment. This issue of how long to treat/run an intervention is therefore vital. However, given the implications for funding interventions, cost-effectiveness has to be a consideration for commissioners and researchers/counsellors running any intervention.

One-year follow-up of measurements in weight-management programmes should perhaps be considered the minimum period for interventions looking for sustained weight-management. This is the inclusion criteria for the National Weight Control Registry in the United States. We propose a minimum of one year's 'treatment' (which includes carrying out measurements as treatment) as an inclusion criterion.

Behavioural Approach

Behaviour change in the context of weight-management often relates to physical activity and nutritional change. The approach, however, for achieving changes clearly differs. Some programmes have a strict prescriptive protocol and the aim is to use behavioural techniques to help participants achieve that prescription. Others focus on facilitating participants who make the decision over what changes they make. Often Behavioural programmes are not based on a specific theory of behaviour (Sharma 2007) and indeed only two we have reviewed.

Weight Loss

Wing and Hill defined a 10% loss of starting weight as a parameter for measuring success (Wing & Hill, 2001) yet they also conclude that >5% of starting body weight is the point at which significant clinical improvement and/or reduction of risk for key lifestyle diseases occurs. As long-term weight loss maintenance is notoriously difficult to achieve, focus on what gains people can make by staying the same weight, losing a little weight and improving key lifestyle indices of health is implicated.

What is a Comprehensive programme?

The criteria for a comprehensive weight-management programme therefore, should include: a minimum treatment period of 1-year, the inclusion of nutrition, physical activity and behaviour change (Perri, 1994, Perri 1986, Soderlund, Fischer & Johansson 2009). Measurements should include: body-composition, bodyweight, dietary-composition, psychological well-being, levels of physical fitness (or amount of participation in physical activity) and dietary changes.

Participants in weight-management programmes might also be usefully convinced of the efficacy of improvements to diet and physical activity *without* weight loss. Although the other factors are deemed important indicators of health protection weight-loss is arguably the primary outcome measure in interventions seeking to improve health this is despite years of data collection demonstrating the extreme difficulty people have in maintaining large amounts of weight loss.

What is success?

Success, therefore, can be defined by improvements to any of the parameters discussed above. Success may include weight loss, but arguably more importantly, body-compositional change, fitness gain, improvement to dietary indices or improvement to general well-being and an increase of confidence in ability to take personal responsibility for personal health. Success perhaps should not relate exclusively to weight loss.

Behavioural Approach across Four Studies

We carried out a systematic review and found four studies which met the *'comprehensive'* criteria discussed above. The model of behaviour change differed from study to study (shown in table 3 below) with one paper simply stating having used a 'behavioural weight loss program' (Cussler et al. 2008) and another describing 'comprehensive behavioural treatment' (Foster et al. 2010) who give examples such as: self-monitoring, stimulus control and relapse management and a clear example of one week's course content for each arm of the low carbohydrate versus low-fat diet. Silva *et al.* (2009) used self-determination theory, which focuses on internalising or making intrinsic motivating factors for carrying out an activity that may have been extrinsic or have externally motivating factors, with the rationale that when the motivation for action is internalised it becomes autonomous and results in favourable outcomes for weight-management. In short when motivation relates to 'doing it for yourself' rather than external factors (the ideally proposed bodyweight, shape etc.) there may be positive outcomes in terms of successful weight-management.

Finally Rapoport, Clark and Wardle (2000) evaluated the use of cognitive behavioural therapy (CBT) modified especially for weight-management (M-CBT) versus a standard CBT (S-CBT). The researchers emphasised a non-dieting approach where instead the focus was on lifestyle change and minimising future weight gain (Rapoport, Clark and Wardle 2000). CBT has an existing evidence base for a range of health problems (Butler, 2006) and takes a variety of approaches including challenging unhelpful thinking and trying out behaviour that may have been previously avoided (Westbrook, 2007).

All studies appeared to follow a semi-prescriptive approach, (to some extent, setting goals determined by the researchers rather than the clients e.g. amount of energy restriction, amount of physical activity) whilst describing tailoring the intervention to the individual's needs. This is a very different to Small Changes where the results are determined by the client facilitated by the trainer.

Table 1 Behavioural approaches

Paper	Behavioural approach
Rapoport , Clark and Wardle (2000)	Cognitive Behavioural Approach
Cussler et al. (2008)	'Comprehensive Behavioural Approach'
Silva et al. (2010)	Self-determination Theory
Foster et al. (2010)	'Behavioural Weight Loss Approach'

Physical Activity Element across the Studies

Physical activity was an element in all the papers we reviewed with approaches varying between a prescription of exactly how much exercise should be done (Rapoport Clark and Wardle, 2000 and Foster et al. 2010 prescribed a specific amount of walking) and measuring what the participants did without indicating that this was promoted/suggested by the programme (Cussler et al. 2008; Silva et al. 2009). All papers described walking as the main mode of exercise.

All of the papers, except Foster et al. (2010), used physical activity questionnaires to assess the duration, (shown below in table 4) type and intensity of physical activity performed and Foster et al. used self-report diaries for participants to record their participation. Walking has previously been described as a 'best buy' in public health terms (Hardman and Stensel p.253, 2003) and seems the most readily repeatable, accessible form of exercise for weight-management programmes. None of the papers discuss alternative modes of physical activity to walking.

Only one paper (Rapoport Clark and Wardle, 2000) measured 'fitness' per se recording lower heart rates at follow-up after repeating a three-minute step test. The other papers recorded increased physical activity participation mostly in the form of increased number of steps. One paper showed a clear relationship between quartile of number of steps and weight loss with those performing least, losing least and those performing most losing most weight and the quartiles in between suggesting a dose response relationship. A comprehensive review suggested that physical activity protects weight regain and may work alone in achieving significant weight loss without diet (Saris et al. 2003).

Table 2. Physical activity measurement

Paper	Physical activity measure
Rapoport , Clark and Wardle (2000)	aerobic fitness via step test and questionnaire on leisure time activity
Cussler et al. (2008)	7-day physical activity recall interview
Silva et al. (2010)	7-day physical activity recall interview
Foster et al. (2010)	self-report diary

Nutrition in the Studies

Only one of the studies reported upon the changes to the quality of subjects' diets (Rapoport Clark and Wardle, 2000). Whereas all attempted to calculate energy intake and changes to calorie intake across the study period, Table 5 highlights the suggested differences between studies. Accurate dietary analysis is notoriously difficult to achieve and subjects are known to under-report intake. Foster et al. (2001), who focussed specifically on following up participants randomised to either a low-carbohydrate diet or a low-fat diet, saw no body-compositional or weight loss differences between the two groups, but more positive blood lipids (and worse side-effects- hair loss, dry mouth, bad breath, constipation) were found in the group consuming a low-carbohydrate diet.

3-day and 7-day diet diaries were used in two studies and the remaining two describe self-reporting. Rapoport et al. (2000) describe detailed nutrient intake, reporting significant reductions in energy consumption, fat intake (both saturated and unsaturated) and sucrose. Similarly there were significant increases in protein and carbohydrate. This data might have been useful across all studies, as dietary improvement may contradict a lack of weight loss.

Table 3 Nutritional assessment

Paper	Nutritional measurement
Rapoport , Clark and Wardle (2000)	Epic Food Frequency Questionnaire (estimated measures)
Cussler et al. (2008)	3-day diet diaries
Silva et al. (2010)	Not measured
Foster et al. (2010)	Difficult to tell, participants 'instructed' to eat 1200-1500 women 1500 to 188 men Kcals a day- no mention of how this was monitored

Weight Loss in the Studies

Table 4 shows the weight loss achieved by each intervention. Across the 4 studies the mean weight loss at one year was around 7% of starting bodyweight. This meets the 5-10% loss of starting weight that can result in substantial reduction of risk from heart disease and type II diabetes (Wing and Hill, 2001). However, the participants' bodyweights at baseline were not the same (neither was BMI) making comparison between studies difficult. The study with participants achieving the greatest weight loss at one year is the study with the heaviest subjects.

The baseline bodyweights of participants in all the studies were a mean of 91.8kgs. BMI ranged from 31 to 36 across the studies.

Table 4. Weight loss

Study	Baseline bodyweight	Weight loss at 1 year
Rapoport , Clark and Wardle (2000)	94 Kg	1.9 kg
Cussler et al. (2008)	84.6Kg	4.6 kg
Silva et al. (2010)	82.1Kg	5.6 kg
Foster et al. (2010)	103.5Kg	7kg

* figures not exact as some of the results are combining two groups e.g. low carb and low fat who had slightly different starting bodyweights and slightly different amounts of weight loss (not statistically significant)

Body-composition Measurements Used in the Studies

There are various methods for measuring body-composition including Dual ex-ray absorptiometry, bio-electrical impedance (BIA) and the gold standard measure under water weighing. Three of the four studies used dual x-ray and BIA for the body-composition analysis. These methods are often used instead of underwater weighing which requires a specialised tank and equipment for analysis and can therefore be prohibitively expensive. Dual x-ray absorptiometry and Bio-electrical impedance have been shown to correlate highly with the under-water weighing method with both obese women (r= 90, p=.001) and healthy weight (r=96, p=.0001) individuals (Erselcan et al. 2000).

Rapoport et al.'s (2000) study used only Waist to Hip Ratio (WHR) to assess body-composition change and found no change in the subjects WHR even though the subjects had lost two kilograms of weight by the end of the programme. Here we must assume that all the weight loss was lean tissue or that the WHR is not sensitive enough to detect such Small Changes to body-composition. The remaining studies all showed loss of lean tissue with around 20-30% of the weight loss coming from lean (NB not all the studies showed statistically significant changes to lean tissue a meta-analysis of results might help determine). There is acceptance of some weight being lost in weight loss programmes coming from lean; however a question arises here over whether protein intake and physical activity should be emphasised or reinforced in an attempt to minimise loss of lean tissue.

A comprehensive programme might pay close attention to the detail of body-composition and attempt to maximise lean tissue protection.

Discussion/Analysis of the Studies

The included studies all found a 'clinically significant' weight loss at ≥1 year i.e. between 5 and 10% of initial weight. However, studies did not all include analysis or discussion around the body-compositional data. Two reported differences in body fat percentage from pre to post-intervention, but did not examine the ratio of fat to lean loss (Cussler et al.,2008, Rapoprt, 2000), while the other two show that ratio (Silva *et al.*, 2010, Foster et al., 2008) . For example, In Silva's study there was a 5.6 kg loss of fat mass and a 1.1 kg loss of lean body mass. In the Foster study 2kg of the 7kg lost was lean tissue. This information should arguably be included in interventions studying weight-management. It is data which adds to our understanding of different interventions and their effects on body-composition/metabolism.

Other work has shown a 80/20 ratio of fat to lean tissue loss, and there may be a protective effect from both physical activity and protein intake on protecting lean tissue during weight loss (Layman et al. 2005). Inclusion of a 'comprehensive' approach to weight-management is implicated. Focus should be on preserving lean tissue and losing fat and not just the objective of fat loss. The focus on fat loss may in fact obfuscate important metabolic/protective results for people who do not lose weight during an intervention, but do make important changes to key indices of health as a result of that intervention (for examples: get fitter increase lean tissue, get better control of blood lipids and blood sugar and increase their score on wellbeing scales). Body-composition and these other measures could be as important as or more important than weight loss.

There are multiple weight-management programmes in the western world being carried out by researchers, health services and in the community. Clearly when the parameters of conducting a comprehensive programme and achieving clinically significant weight loss, as outlined by Wing and Hill (2001), are employed, the programmes that have been scrutinised in this review are successful in meeting both criteria.

The problem of overweight is widely considered to relate to nutrition and physical activity and people's behaviour in relation to these. Approaches that include all three of these elements are sufficient in length to gain maximum effect and consider key measurements of health (not just weight) have been analysed for this review.

However, an outstanding further consideration for debate for public health interventions is cost-effectiveness. There doesn't seem to be inclusion of this in any of the papers reviewed here. The solutions sought by public health providers need this element including so that commissioners are able to assess not only how robust the approach is but also whether it can be paid for. Often interventions run on research grants or money from the public purse. This begs the question: if we do identify and agree upon what success is and how it is achieved, can we afford to pay for it?

Body-composition is an important element of weight loss programmes; indeed focus on weight loss alone is negative as it belies the other key parameters that may proffer protection for health as mentioned above. Using an equation, such as the one proposed here, that identifies both negative and positive weight loss and maximising strategies to preserve lean tissue whilst losing fat tissue will be useful. The inclusion of comprehensive content, exercise, nutrition, a behavioural approach and sufficient follow-up are all included in comprehensive interventions.

Future work

In the field of weight-management, the inclusion of a comprehensive programme and clearly agreed measures of success needs augmenting with cost-effectiveness data. What use is the most effective, comprehensive programme if it cannot be paid for?

Summary

Discussion around what represents a comprehensive weight-management programme could reasonably conclude that the key features are the inclusion of nutrition/food, physical activity *and* a clear element of behaviour change (Soderlund, 2009; Peri et al. 1984). These ingredients should also be augmented by a reasonable period of treatment/monitoring so that not only weight loss but also maintenance of weight loss is included (Perri et al. 1989), with realistic goal setting as part of the approach (NICE guidelines, 2006).

Chapter 2 Assessment

These 5 key questions will help clarify your understanding of the key components in a successful weight-management programme

1. What are the three proposed essential components in a successful weight-management programme?

2. What seems to be the ideal (realistic) length of time for running a programme?

3. Which measures would you make in your programme to detect body-compositional change rather than just weight loss?

4. What else, besides weight loss and body-composition changes, would be an example of a positive outcome in a weight-management programme?

5. Give a valid criticism to a programme that produces findings showing weight loss and positive change at 10-20 weeks

Answers in Appendix 1

References

BACON et al. (2005) Size Acceptance and Intuitive Eating Improve Health for Obese, Female Chronic Dieters *J Am Diet Assoc.*;**105**:929-936

BAZZANO et al. (2008) Intake of Fruit, Vegetables, and Fruit Juices and Risk of Diabetes in Women Diabetes Care, **31**,(7), 1311-1317

BOOIL J (2002) Statistical Power in Randomized Intervention Studies With Noncompliance *Psychological Methods* **7**,(2), 178-193

BOUCHARD C (1990) The Response to Long-term Overfeeding in Identical Twins N Engl J Med, **322**:1477-1482

BRECKON, J. JOHNSON, L.H. and HUTCHISON, A. (2008). Physical Activity   Counseling Content and Competency: A Systematic Review. *Journal of Physical Activity and Health,* **5**, 398-417.

BUTLER AC, et al. (January 2006). 'The empirical status of cognitive-behavioral therapy: a review of meta-analyses'. *Clin Psychol Rev* **26** (1): 17–31.

CASP tools online http://www.sph.nhs.uk/what-we-do/public-health-workforce/resources/critical-appraisals-skills-programme last accessed December 2010

CUSSLER E.C, et al. (2008) Maintenance of Weight Loss in Overweight Middle-aged Women through the Internet. *Obesity,* **16**, (5), 1052-1060

DEPARTMENT OF HEALTH (2010) *Health Survey for England 2008* the Stationary office London.

ERSELCAN, T et al. (2000) Comparison of body-composition analysis methods in clinical routine. *Annals of Nutrition and Metabolism,* **44**(5-6) 243-248

FORESIGHT (2007) Tackling Obesities: Future Choices Government Office for Science. http://www.bis.gov.uk/foresight/our-work/projects/current-projects/tackling-obesities/reports-and-publications

FOSTER et al. (2010) Weight and metabolic Outcomes After 2 Years on a Low-Carbohydrate Versus Low-Fat Diet *Ann Int Med* **153**:147-157

FOX, K (1999) The Influence of physical activity on mental well-being *Public Health Nutrition* **2** (3a), 411-418

FRIED, L. et al.. (2001)Frailty in older adults: evidence for a pheno-type. *J Gerontol.*:**56A**, M146 –56.

GUYATT G.H, Sackett DL and Cook DJ (1993) Users' guides to the medical literature *JAMA* **270**,(21),2598-2601

GUYATT, G.H, Sackett DL and Cook DJ (1994) How to use an article about therapy or prevention. *JAMA* **271**,(1),59-63

HARDMAN A, Stensel D (2003) Physical Activity and Health the Evidence Explained Routledge, London

JANSEN I, Heymsfield, S.B , Ross, R (2002) Low Relative Skeletal Muscle Mass (Sarcopenia) in Older Persons Is Associated with Functional Impairment and Physical Disability *Journal of the American Geriatrics Society* **50**,(5), 889-896

LAYMAN et al. (2005) Dietary Protein and Exercise have Additive Effects on body-composition During Weight Loss in Adult Women *J.Nutr* **135**, 1903-1910

MHURCHU, C.N. Margetts, B.M. Speller, V. (1998) Randomized clinical control trial comparing the effectiveness of two dietary interventions for patients with hyperlipidemia *Clinical Science*. 95, 479-487

MILLER, W.R. (1983) Motivational interviewing with problem drinkers. *Behavioural Psychotherapy*, 11, 147-172.

NATIONAL INSTITUTE for HEALTH and CLINICAL EXCELLENCE (2006) Obesity: the prevention, identification, assessment and management of overweight and obesity in adults and children http://guidance.nice.org.uk/CG43

NATIONAL WEIGHT CONTROL REGISTRY http://www.nwcr.ws/default.htm *last accessed 21.01.10*

NISHIDA et al. (2004) The Joint WHO/FAO Expert Consultation on diet, nutrition and the prevention of chronic diseases: process, product and policy implications. *Public Health Nutrition*: 7(1A), 245–250

PAFFENBARGER et al. (1986) Physical Activity, All-cause Mortality and Longevity of College Alumni *N Engl J Med* **314**, 605-613

PERRI ,M.G. et al. (1984) Effect of a multicomponent maintenance program on long-term weight loss *Journal of Consulting and Clinical Psychology* 52, 3, 480-481

PERRI M G. Et al. (1989) Effect of length of treatment on weight loss. *Journal of Consulting and Clinical Psychology*, **57** (3), 450-452.

PRENTICE A.M, Jebb S.A (1995) Obesity in Britain gluttony or sloth? BMJ 311:437

RAPOPORT L, Clark M, Wardle J (2000) Evaluation of a modified cognitive-behavioural programme for weight-management International *Journal of Obesity*, **24**, 1726-1737

ROUBENOFF R, Hughes V. (1997) Sarcopenia: current concepts. J *Gerontol: Med Sci.*;**55A**:M716 –24.

SARIS et al. (2003) How much physical activity is enough to prevent unhealthy weight gain? Outcome of the IASO 1st Stock Conference and consensus statement obesity reviews **4**,101–114

SATI MAZUMDAR et al. (1999) Intent-to-treat analysis for longitudinal clinical trials: coping with the challenge of missing values *Journal of Psychiatric Research* **33**, 87-95

SHARMA (2007) Behavioural interventions for preventing and treating obesity in adults. *Obesity reviews* **8**, 441-449

SILVA et al. (2010) Using self-determination theory to promote physical activity and weight control: a randomized controlled trial in women *J Behav Med*, **33**: 110-122

SMITH-WEST, D. et al. (2007). Motivational interviewing Improves Weight Loss in Women With Type 2 Diabetes, *Diabetes Care*, 30; 5, 1081-1087.

SODERLUND. A, Fischer. A, Johannson, T (2009) Physical activity, diet and behaviour modification in the treatment of overweight and obese adults: a systematic review Perspectives in Public Health **129**(3)132-142

SURGEON General report (1996) Physical Activity and Health: A Report of the Surgeon General, Centers for Disease Control and Prevention, Atlanta

VAN DORSTEN B (2007) The Use of Motivational Interviewing in Weight loss *Current Diabetes Reports* 7:386-390

WADDEN et al. (2009) One-year Weight Losses in the Look AHEAD Study: Factors Associated With Success *Obesity* **17**,(4), 713-722

WADDEN et al. (1992) Clinical Correlates of short- and long-term weight loss *Am J Clin Nutr* **56**, 271s-4s

WING, R.R,HILL J.O (2001) Successful Weight Loss Maintenance *Annual Review of Nutrition* **21**: 323-341

WARE J.H, (2003) Interpreting Incomplete Data in Studies of Diet and Weight Loss *NEJM* **348**, (21), 2136-2137

WESTBROOK D, Kennerly H, Kirk J (2007) An Introduction to Cognitive Behavioural Therapy: Skills and Applications Sage London

CHAPTER 3

RAISING AWARENESS

Chapter Objectives

- To give examples of awareness raising techniques

- To recognise barriers and responses to change

Questioning:

Asking the client useful, non-threatening questions is an art. This skill lies in the questioner's motive. Our focus with Small Changes is to ask questions to which the client needs an answer. Our motive is to raise the client's self-awareness, much less often are we actually seeking information for ourselves.

Questions that can be answered only with 'yes' or 'no' are closed questions. They solicit information that the questioner wants to hear and they can also indicate the direction that the questioner wants them to take.

e.g. *'Did you tell your brother that you had crashed his car?'*

There are only two answers to this question and the client knows both of them. They can of course elucidate, but if they do not offer more information, we need to ask in a different way.

e.g. *'How did you feel when you were planning to tell your brother about the crash?'*

This is an open question that allows the client to explore her reactions to the situation and become more aware of underlying fear, shame, withdrawal, deceit, anger or other responses to stress.

The facilitator can ask a question without asking a question. To encourage a participant to say more ask them to repeat the last detail they gave you with an upward tone at the end which suggests your statement could be a question.

e.g. *'I see. You are thinking that your mother will make an embarrassing comment in front of your friends?'*

This is a statement that uses their words to underline what the participant has just said, but it sounds like a question. The participant will hear it as a question or they will agree with your summary and add more details. In either case they are still paying attention to the possible embarrassment and becoming aware of how significant it is to them.

With this awareness clients are able to decide how to safely challenge themselves and then take the action of their choice.

Evaluation

Using a drawing of a mountain, or a tree, clients are asked to mark the place they feel represents their health when the top of the mountain or tree is considered optimal in relation to their weight/health. This can be measured again half way through a programme and at the end and even though reaching the top or 'optimal' is unlikely in even a long programme clients can (and do in our experience) see themselves making progress.

A rating scale of 1- 5, one being low/little and five being high/huge can be used for self-evaluation of confidence, ability, motivation or any criteria that the client needs to take into account when making a change. A 1 – 10 scale is an alternative, but this is often familiar to clients from school days and other situations where ten was regarded as perfect. Only a minority of people will rate themselves or their situations as perfect and the amount of numbers before ten may offer too many positions for a facilitator to clearly understand where the client feels she stands. So we have settled on a 1-5 scale as easier for facilitator and client.

It is vital to pose questions to which the client needs an answer. This will raise their awareness of how important the issue they are talking about feels to them. They may say it is a high priority because it is affecting their daily life so badly that they need to do something about it immediately. They may say it rates a 4 on a scale of 1 -5 for example.

A facilitator might want to check if there is any other issue that is as, or more pressing, that will get in the way, by asking if other current issues are at 4 or higher. A spouse in hospital, an exam in the next week, debt, truanting children, a sick pet, may all be rated higher, because they are more immediate or overwhelming, for the client at this time.

In motivational interviewing a key idea with scaling questions is to focus on the positive – for example:

SC: *'How confident do you feel about this on a scale of 1 to 5 with 5 being absolutely sure and 1 being really unconfident'.*

Client: '2'

SC: 'O*K so you're a 2 and not a 0. How come you're that confident?'.*

Here what is happening is the counsellor avoids the 'trap' of responding with 'Oh you're only a 2 why not higher?' Which MI counsellors will tell you is likely to lead to the client listing all the negative reasons as to why their confidence is low. Whereas, by focusing on being higher than a 0 - the client is then likely to list all the factors which *do* give them confidence.

Time

Available time is a persistent issue. Change demands time within the context of a life that is already assigned. All activities need to be measured in order to see where a change can be made.

A circle is divided into quarters representing the 24 of hours in a day/night. Each section represents six hours. Activity can be measured by colouring hours spent sleeping, lying down and sitting time – sedentary jobs, reading, meals - in red. These are the hours of non-activity, of sitting and lying down. Rising to make a cup of tea during TV advertisements is not counted as activity!

Yellow represents time spent on your feet, moving – gardening, shopping, cleaning, ironing – any activity that excludes sitting or lying down.

Green represents exercise from brisk walking to hiking and mountaineering and anything in between. Sports, training, attending the gym, swimming and aqua-aerobics, Ballroom to Zumba dancing – any activity that raises the heart rate, induces sweating or prevents singing due to breathlessness.

When completed the circle shows it's owner exactly where most time is spent, how often activities are useful/healthy and how many hours they feel are 'wasted'. It gives client's the information they need in order to assign time to chosen changes. These may be an increase of time already used yellow and green, or a change that reduces red.

Food Diary

Divide a table into seven days across and 24 hours down, with the hours sectioning the 24 hours to delineate breakfast, elevenses, lunch, afternoon snack, evening meal, supper, night-time fridge raids. The diary should reflect the cultural norms of the clients. There should be enough space for the client to note when and what they ate, but not how much. Try and ensure that they can make a habit of keeping this simple diary every day. Check for `grazing' between meals and snacks.

The overall general picture will indicate the type of meals and snacks eaten, the distribution throughout the week and the times they do not eat. It raises awareness of life-long choices, habits and unquestioned attitudes of '*I always...I never*'eat. Assure those who excuse themselves by declaring that one day was '*not an unusual day and therefore does not count'* these unusual days occur all the time in our experience – this is real life! e.g. unexpected visitors, visiting family in hospital, tummy aches, attending conferences, weddings, holidays and all other celebrations or traditions such as Pancake Tuesday.

Label reading

Cards the size of credit cards listing the levels of fat, salt and sugar that are low, medium and high, can be used by for clients to rate their regularly purchased, packaged food items. The shock of their individual findings is often enough to promote changes to other brands with reduced amounts, to substitute other ingredients or buy fresh fruit and vegetables and ingredients to cook from scratch.

Clients usually ask for more information about what they are 'supposed to do'. Government recommendations are often too big a leap, therefore Small Changes can be encouraged e.g. aiming for a shopping trolley with 75% of items in the 'medium' yellow range, as many in the green, fresh, 'low' fat, salt and sugar as possible and if there are a couple of items in the 'high' red range -, enjoy them.

The first day shopping with a card will take twice as long and be ten times more memorable than any other. The awareness gained cannot be erased without more effort than it takes to continue health threatening consumption.

Portion sizes

The NHS Eatwell Plate shows the comparative amounts of meat, vegetables/fruit and dairy which that are advised for the general public. If clients bring their usual main meal plate and breakfast bowl they can compare their current portion sizes. By using food or substitutes, for instance a pack of cards to represent a portion of meat, as recommended by the British Heart Foundation, the physical interaction of increasing or reducing the remembrance of what constitutes a portion is more likely to be retained.

A participant in this session piled his plate with the artificial vegetables and potatoes, adding three packs of cards to represent his usual intake of meat. When asked about the meat, he confidently described it as lean and not fried. As we moved on to look at the plates of other participants, the man interrupted.

Pointing out the two, or one pack of cards on the plates of other participants, he commented 'They don't eat much do they!' He removed one pack of cards from his plate when the recommended size of meat portion was explained to him.

He half wanted to follow the recommendation and half to continue enjoying a portion two thirds too large. The decision to try eating only twice as much as recommended was an effective start leading to a further reduction by the end of the course.

The individual experiences of education, parental control, stress, convenience, grazing, shared family habits, have already played a part in the life of individual people and it is these particular factors that obese clients first need to become aware of in relation to themselves.

An awareness of the personal effect that the level of individual education an individual has received may restrict their access to any presentation of information or facilities is a vital component of change. Lack of opportunity and parental care may shrink s personal boundaries to the point where it is difficult to find an internal locus of control.

Parental Control

A lack of opportunity to make personal decisions, or close parental care, may shrink personal boundaries to the point where it is difficult to find an internal locus of control.

Although clients are generally able to examine in detail, the style of parental control in their own childhood home, they may be unaware of the precise effect it had in the formation of their character. Referring to their memories of what were normal, accepted events and relationships at home, a mature client has the opportunity to explore memories and reactions from an adult position. As their awareness increases, clients are able to reassess and alter their present attitudes and actions - to decide for themselves..

A really good key example of this, and one that frequently comes up frequently in Small Changes, relates to 'clearing your plate'. Clients will say we were taught to always clear our plates. There seems to be a sense here of not wasting food and how negative it seems to throw food away. One of our clients later juxtaposed their original thoughts by saying 'better in the bin than in you'. They were not promoting the wastage of food but merely recognising that early messages may now be outdated. The conclusion is of course, to prepare smaller portions.

Stress Awareness

An awareness of the cause and effect of stress is crucial to a client's ability to accommodate changes within the context of their lives. The major difficulty for most clients is to craft a space for themselves, while still fulfilling their obligations to family, friends and employers.

One person's stress is another's drive, but the common factor is how these are affecting their lives in terms of personal health and well-being. The barrier that the greatest number of clients experience, is an inability to put self first, even it is vital to carve out fifteen minutes to attend to their own needs. Free time seems an impossible dream. Raising awareness of the ultimate effect of continuing under stress, or the possibility that taking care of their own needs will not having a damaging effect on those for whom they are responsible, affords a client the freedom to consider and choose from the available options.

Raising Awareness with a Food Diary

Clients usually know the difference between grazing and meals, although those who profess to eat 'nothing' all day are often constantly grazing. They do not count any food swallowed when standing up, or not using a knife and fork, as 'eating'. Awareness of the individual extent of the grazing factor on obesity is gained in the early stages of a Small Changes course. Grazing is often mostly a habit stimulated by boredom, and or ingrained habit, or psychological trauma. In cases where the shortage of food meant that people had to eat what and when they could, the stimulus to consume food may be constant. Raising an awareness of periods of boredom, generally promotes activity and this change of habit reduces the time when unconscious grazing takes place.

We very often find that client's awareness of eating patterns is immediately raised by keeping a diet diary. This need not be exact with precise amounts, but merely a representation of the types of things people eat, the number of times a day they eat and of course missing meals.

A Typical Day

The baseline of 'Small Changes' approach to working with an individual is not what we want to hear about, but what the participant wants to think about. Information is given on request, ensuring that clients only have to attend to information that is specific to them and relevant to the issue with which they are dealing. Our status quo is that the clients are in charge of their individual lives. They will set the best direction for them to take, at any given point of time. The absence of direction from a facilitator avoids upsetting this status quo. The client is the expert. They are safeguarded from suspecting that the facilitator knows best, trying to please them, or becoming dependent.

It is vital to ask questions to which the client needs an answer. This will raise the participant's awareness of how important to them is the issue they are talking about. They may say it is a high priority, because it is effecting their daily lives so badly that they need to do something about it immediately. They may say it rates a 9 on a scale of 1 -10. An often used technique is to ask the client to explain a typical day. This allows the client to reflect on how they spend their time, what and when they eat etc.

Elaboration

Encouraging a client to say more can be achieved by using summary and reflection techniques. The facilitator can use a pause in the client's story, or indicate to the client that she wants to speak, which avoids speaking over the client or interrupting.

Summarising involves playing back the last few sentences the client has spoken. e.g.:

SC: *'Let me get this right... after you fell, some of the shoppers tried to help, but you were so upset you could not tell them about losing your purse?'*

The client takes this opportunity to calm herself and then continues to relate the details of the mugging, her injuries and loss of money and how she is now too afraid to leave her house without an escort.

Reflecting back to the client the story she is telling, or the feelings she is experiencing, affords the client reassurance that she is being carefully listened to and gives her the confidence to look more deeply into the issues. Facilitator making a simple reflection relating to an event:

SC: *'I can understand that after such a long time gap, a letter telling you about Jane was a complete surprise.'*

Facilitator making a complex reflection relating to feelings:

SC: '*You feel totally confused about your reactions, like your initial excitement and joy at knowing that Jane was well and wanting to see you again, was mixed up with fury. Now you are wondering if you actually hate her and whether you want to see her again.* '

There are always reasons behind any failure to succeed in making a small change. Present and past life often gets in the way with contrary demands. Had we explored beyond Ellen's enjoyment of swimming as a child and looked more closely at the gap between then and now, Ellen would have become aware of how difficult it would be to go near deep water having spent two days in a coma at the age of eight after almost drowning.

Previous experiences, successes or failures, will influence the participant. Their memories may produce a heightened expectancy of success or an inappropriate fear of failure. Assisting the participant to explore these past experiences will raise their awareness of the significance and possible effect on their attitudes today. Reflecting back to the participant the words they have chosen to describe experiences is a simple way of allowing them to hear their thoughts out loud a second time, which can lead to more insights. Reflecting on the emotions that their narratives arouses is a more complex, but also an effective approach for the participant.

Drawing together the main details that the participant is exploring in a summary, also allows them to hear their words again, with the added bonus of knowing that they have been listened to. This increases the rapport that has been established and will have a positive effect on the participant's confidence in their sovereignty.

Why don't people just change?

Is there any other issue that has so massively engaged so many individuals? They know, but why do they not act? It does not make sense until we take into account the factors that may prevent people from responding to good, simple advice.

The notion that eating (poorly) drinking (too much) alcohol smoking (anything) and not exercising are behaviours we carry out simply because we are blasé about the health risks is perhaps implausible. Instead it might be that these are simply poor decisions, made quickly and in response to positive feedback. Take for an example, the decision to stop smoking, we might make this decision as it reduces health-risk, improves income and personal aroma. These are logical rationale to change- the feedback from health-risk and income will take some time to appear - weeks to months. If we compare this to feeling stressed or walking into a bar where the atmosphere and sights, sounds smells remind us how good we will immediately feel after a cigarette you can see the problem.

So there is a distance between the positive feedback and the behaviour and essentially of course we all we make quick and slow decisions. We need to make quick decisions all the time (think crossing the road) but we don't want to make all decisions quickly! Perhaps decisions on how we live, the amount we eat, whether we ever relax or not, who we propose to or don't should be made somewhat slower than crossing the road. As I leave the train station each morning I am assailed by the aroma of freshly baked pastries and cafe latte - this aroma emanates from a cleverly positioned vendor at the exit to my platform. I want to control my weight, be slim and keep fit and these things will all happen with regular exercise and restricted amounts of calories and alcohol (in my experience) however if I am overweight these things take weeks and months to give feedback (quite slow but very powerful once experienced). The pastry and latte give immediate feedback- yum.

Food and exercise decisions might be better made slowly and thought through, which in turn might mean counsellors are useful when we are deciding whether to change or not. I will, of course, be the one to decide what I do day by day, the counsellor might just help me get there.

The question why don't people just change? Applies to much behaviour, why am I not organised enough? Why don't I save money? (These two behaviours apply to Jean and Trevor). The answer will rely on feedback e.g. saving equals benefits much later but I can see a brand new pair of shoes I want now! And organisation would be great because I will find all the papers in place later when I come to look for them but it is very convenient to just put them down here right now...

There are other reasons for not 'just changing' for example communities who do not have access to fresh fruit and vegetables, or sufficient space in their fridge freezers to take enough frozen products to feed a larger family. Tight budgets are an issue alongside historically established likes and dislikes. The lack of cooking experience - what do you do with a kohlrabi? How do you hack into a butternut squash? Can everyone afford a steamer? And above all else, the kids won't touch it.

Understanding how we came to establish our likes and dislikes, our whole relationship to food, not just what we eat, but why we eat, it might help us change. If we explore how clients copied their parents, responded to situations of too much easily available food or shortages of basic foods; treat, comfort or defend themselves with food; eat without noticing; do not recognise or respond to appetite signals; then people might be able to make effective healthy changes. They can answer that question 'Just what does get in your way?'

If the target were tailored to fit each individual, they would be able to imagine how to reach it. To eat one, only one more portion of fruit, or vegetable, which may already be eaten regularly, is an achievable target. It only challenges the insufficient amount of food, not tastes or habits, or the autonomy of an individual. Achieving that target results in personal confidence and insight and a desire to do more is established.

Schemes that encourage healthy eating

That instruction to 'eat healthily' is now buttressed by information leaflets emphasising the desirable effects. This campaign to change the national lack of awareness has been taken up by individuals and communities. Grow Your Own projects together with shops concentrating on locally grown produce, are co-operating with Incredible Edible town schemes. People are gaining skills, enjoying Cook and Eat classes, practising the skills at home and absorbing a plethora of information in magazines, newspapers and supermarkets. From local cafes and restaurants, to major supermarkets and fast food franchise chains, the pressure of the 'healthy option' is virtually impossible to avoid.

A major home furnishing company is giving employees free lunches if they choose the store's own restaurant healthy option (which is also at a lower price for customers). Jamie Oliver (a celebrity chef in the United Kingdom) tackled school head teachers and their dinner ladies and is now training young chefs. Private sector slimming clubs are funded with vouchers handed to patients by GP practices. The NHS and town councils have been putting money into schemes that reach the least resourced local communities.

Television programmers confront us with the spectacle of other people, including those in the highest risk category of morbidly obese, undergoing the most extraordinarily punishing exercise programmes. This is as near to watching death defying high wire circus trapeze acts as we can get. Rigid with the tension of anticipating a fall, we are relieved that no-one dies. Boot Camp programmes court the same risk and we are surprised that the participants survive. It is the companies that need to advertise drink products and food to enormous audiences that fund these shows. The inference is that their brand is healthier than their competitors' brand and is produced by people who are making a committed effort to improve the health of the nation.

Football clubs are luring men into the stadiums, giving them access to nutritional information, fitness training time with coaches and football games. Individuals are taking part in local walking groups, exercise in the park sessions, and personalised gym programmes. Swimming baths with aquaerobic and women only sessions, tennis clubs, five-a-side football clubs and dancing classes, have attracted huge numbers of people who gave up exercise and sport years ago. From strolling on the canal tow paths to 'come when you can' boot camp sessions in the park, there are now more opportunities to be active at whatever level is appropriate.

It could be argued that awareness at the community and general population level has been successfully raised. Indeed many people have lost weight and yet still the weight lost often finds its way back. In our, and others, experience the weight is often regained with 'interest'. There is little doubt we are collectively unhappy about weight- some of us about our own weight and some others who are worried about the weight of others, Patients and clients for examples.

Why Information alone is not enough

Half way through a Small Changes course, a participant who had lost 10lbs and was feeling very pleased with her newly found energy and confidence, commented: *'I just needed to know what to eat and what not to eat. When I am shopping now, my mind tells me 'Oh no, that is not healthy,' so I choose a healthy option.'*

How did she miss the ubiquitous messages?

Fresh vegetables and fruit, lean meat, oily fish, salads – YES; takeaways, fast food, high fat, sugar, salt content – NO.

She did not miss the messages. She simply thought that they did not apply to her. No-one thinking about joining a Small Changes course has ever answered the question 'Do you eat healthily?' with a 'No'.

We all have the desire and ability to be responsible for our own health status. We also have difficulty in sorting out the propaganda from authentic guidance. Our choice of food has been mitigated by what we were used to in childhood, our level of income, accessibility, our cooking skills, culture, insufficient knowledge and pure basic habit.

Faced with this compelling evidence, Small Changes had to conclude that all the information, facilities, rewards, threats, free activity tickets and encouragement are still not enough.

If the general publicity, information and guidance on how to improve health and reduce obesity is comprehensive, accessible and of a high standard – why are we not seeing a significant reduction in the numbers of people becoming obese What have we missed? The answer may be – the variable human being.

Each person is unique in their experience of life. No two people have totally the same experience or reaction, no matter how similar their up-bringing and life events are. Their personal narrative is just that – personal. It is reflected in their understanding and attitudes, their motives, morals and values.

When we exclaim 'Oh, that's just you!' we are saying that we recognise the person's reasoning, and fully expect it, because we know how she reasons and behaves. We know who and how she is. If the people that we know well behave in an unexpected way we feel surprised. The deviation from their norm is worrying and even frightening.

The personal narrative highlights what each individual considers to be the most important factors in his or her life – at any given moment in time. The life of each human being consists of a unique combination of factors that are fluid. Experiences, circumstances and age add to the personal narrative and influence both minor and major changes.

We simply cannot provide one route to health covering everyone. Nor can *we* ever know all that there is to know, about someone else. That 'someone else' knows everything about themselves. It is from this position that Small Changes chose to make raising the awareness of participants one of the key factors of our approach. Given the opportunity to remember all they know, people can use the information to make changes that will endure.

This means we recognise that every participant has all the facts that they personally need to take into consideration, when planning to assume responsibility for their own well-being. It also means we recognise that people are interested in and capable of, taking charge of their own health. The person is not the problem; the problem is the problem (White 2007).

Small Changes and client sovereignty (*sovereign: supreme ruler*)

The client is autonomous. Small Change clients choose their priorities, make decisions on how to begin making changes and then follow through with the appropriate actions. The course facilitator's first step is to enable the clients to raise their personal, unique awareness. In other words the client has ownership or *sovereignty* over their own issue of change.

By reviewing the factors that contributed to their choice of lifestyle, their discomfort or contentment with the results, each person will be facilitated to consider the changes they feel they need to make. These changes have a scale of precedence for the client. The one that takes priority is not necessarily the most vital or most important in losing weight. Nor may it be the first change a client considers, or the one that seems the easiest or the most terrifying.

The 'Right It' reflex

A potential problem, perhaps for people working in health and social care, is the drive to fix people's problems. What we are actually suggesting is to be aware of the *right it* reflex (a phrase used by Miller and Rollnick in their motivational interviewing work) and rather than act on it support the client's right to own their own problems.

Case Study: weight gain linked to bereavement

A mother grieving for her adult son, who committed suicide, and struggling with his widow's refusal to allow her to see the two grandchildren, joined a Small Changes group when her weight started to increase as she ate for comfort.

It may be obvious that the teacakes loaded with butter do not assist weight loss. If she took advice to cut out the teacakes, she would also be cutting out her defence against despair. The loss of her son, not being able to see her grandchildren and the collapse of P's relationship with her daughter-in-law, were the most pressing issues in her life.

After those issues, she worried about her increasing weight. Given support to examine the whole situation and repair it, P regained time with her grandchildren and increased her activity by having them stay at her house at weekends, playing in the park and going for regular swims.

Often it is the most desired change that comes to mind immediately the question is asked.

*'What would you like to change in your life, that would make you healthier and happier - if you could choose anything that is **reasonably** possible?'* This question is constructed to safeguard the client from the disappointment. Realising, often with humour, that some imagined changes are just not possible given their current life situation just as growing hair on a bald head or dancing the lead role in Swan Lake are unlikely if not impossible.

After the desired area of change is disclosed, the attention moves onto how important this area is to them when compared with other changes in other areas that they would like to tackle.

On a scale of one to five, one being low and five being high, we ask the client how important is the need for the suggested change? If a figure below five is chosen, this first area of change may need to be put to one side and another area chosen for comparison. Whichever is the participant's highest priority can be successfully tackled first, which will increase the likelihood that other issues worked on later will not be abandoned in favour of the most important issue.

As self-awareness increases, the ability to see more of their personal 'Big Picture' also increases. The client will be able to suggest a change and after considering the things that may get in her way, rate her confidence in accomplishing it. Awareness of people, lack of time, acting alone, or any other issue that could impede her success, creates an opportunity to avoid or manage these difficulties.

In order to accurately pinpoint what they want to achieve and to imagine the various ways they might successfully use, clients need to examine how and why they arrived at this point, this situation in their lives. There are obstacles preventing them making the change. Were this not so, the change would have been easily made perhaps a long time ago. Support will be needed, from verbal encouragement to physical presence, to ensure and witness the change and the results.

Conclusions from a case study

The Small Changes approach does not direct or guide a participant. Examination of life experience, talk of present lifestyle and remembrance of past success, is fundamental. Facilitators listen with 100% attention as clients recognise the fears and pressures that influence their choices. It is essential that the clients listen to themselves. The narrative in all its detail is infinitely more vital for the client to hear than the facilitator.

The participant does all the work of assessing what they want to achieve; the facilitator maintains the position and conveys to the client in words or attitude, that every decision they have made was the best possible decision, given the information and choices that were available to them at the time.

By composing an internal picture in the mind, the past is moved into the present. Clients recall incidental or 'forgotten' memories, which are rarely recalled because they were the ordinary fabric of their lives. These unremarkable patterns of bedtimes, mealtimes, school timetables, parental control and care, are filed in long-term memory. Recollection as mature adults renders an understanding of the ethnicity of a person's current lifestyle.

Piloted to self-knowledge, a client is able to understand through amplification of their narrative, how each factor contributes to their present day values. The path to current habits is laid down from birth. Everyone feels it to be 'me'. This 'me' is accepted and felt as authentic, as a true and a freely self-directed human being.

To challenge a client's version of self is a delicate and serious matter. A well-meant suggestion or an inattentive comment on a client's attitude or decisions, can have a catastrophic effect. In an effort to live through and beyond past events or traumatic experiences, the kind that form or deform a person, we defend ourselves from feelings experienced at the time of the event or trauma.

The human brain has been described as a tape recorder. We may 'forget' experiences and be unable to bring them to mind, but they are still recorded for eternity in the brain. Along with events, the brain also records any associated feelings. Both feelings and events stay locked together and when replayed, occluded experiences are vivid. They effect how we feel at the time of replaying. (Penfold, 1975) This re-experiencing of past traumatic events may result in a re-living, which amounts to going through the experience as though it was the first time.

There is always, without exception, a reason for defences constructed as children, adolescents or adults. Breaching these defences will expose the person to the earlier trauma, which they may then re-live and feel as though it happened two seconds ago. The original reactions, whether demonstrated or suppressed at the time, will return.

Forgotten incidents may be so obscured from consciousness that the resulting defensive behaviour is not recognised as defensive.

Case study : a past factor

Three weeks after deciding to go swimming with a friend, Ellen still had not made this 'small' change. The first week she found her swimming costume had holes in it and her shopping day was the day after her swimming date.

The second week she was feeling tired through losing sleep with a nightmare.

On the third week Ellen forgot the time and missed the bus. Obviously the exploration of this choice of a small change had not been quite thorough enough. It was necessary to go beyond the fact that she could swim and had enjoyed it as a child; that she always enjoyed being out with her friend; that she had time to go swimming and a costume to wear. It was such a good idea. Other people in the group swam every week and came in with animated tales of the fun they had had together.

SC: '*Who did you swim with as a child Ellen?* '

Ellen: '*The usual gang, kids living in our neighbourhood, we used to have a great time in the river. There were about nine of us, noisy crowd!* '

SC: '*It sounds as though you enjoyed being outside with those noisy friends?* '

Ellen: '*Yes.* ' Long pause.

'*Till I nearly drowned.... I was eight years old. Mam told me I was unconscious for two days. I haven't been swimming since then.* '

She never did swim again.

This is one example of a typical way that people sometimes choose to make a change, in any area of behaviour. At the start of the course we may encourage them to choose past enjoyable experiences, or to join a friend for support. In Ellen's case she was carried along by the enthusiasm of the group and only remembered happy childhood times in the river. Even if she had remembered drowning, she may not have anticipated a problem. Nor did she connect the reasons for not going swimming for three weeks, with that early trauma.

Defences range from eating or not eating, health threatening increases or decreases of weight, addictions, rigid adherence to habit, likes and dislikes, personality traits, to could-have-been dreams and plans that were never acted upon. The issue with defences is that they are often maintained beyond their purpose. They are no longer needed, but have become rigidities that prevent growth and freedom of choice.

Stages of Change

The stage of change or transtheoretical model (TTM) was first proposed by Prochaska and Diclemente 1980. The TTM suggests that in relation to change we are all in one of a number of stages – these are:

- Pre-contemplation
- Contemplation
- Preparation
- Action
- Maintenance
- Relapse

In Pre-contemplation I am not thinking about or considering change. Contemplation maybe typified by the attitude 'I really ought to do something about this...'. Preparation is for example the point at which I go to the shop and buy some training shoes. Action is the initial period when I start jogging. Maintenance is most often talked about as the point where I've been carrying out the behaviour (or stopping the behaviour i.e. Smoking), for six months or so.

Is relapse a failure, or Just a Stage of Change?

Relapse is where I revert back to doing or not doing the target behaviour. Interestingly relapse is seen as a normal part of long term success – for example – smokers seem to stop smoking a mean average of 4 times before the change becomes a permanent one.

Small Changes techniques

Without awareness of the origins, clients are unable to change habits that inhibit healthy changes. The Small Changes approach enables people to raise their awareness of the source of the problems that influence them and their significant relationships. It is more productive to focus on the effects on people's lives, rather than on the problems. It is more effective to reflect upon and connect with their intentions, values, hopes and commitments and to applaud the strength and resilience people have shown in resistance to problem pressures.

3 Assessment

1. Raising awareness is a matter of showing the client where they are going wrong? T or F

2. Raising awareness allows the client to decide what is happening in a given situation and to use the information to help them make decisions T or F

3. Acceptance of the client's narrative is absolutely key in behaviour change. T or F

4. Relapsing into old habits denotes the client's lack of will power? T or F

Answers in Appendix 1

References

BERNE E. 1964., Games People Play. USA. Grove
Press/Random House, USA

Foresight Project Director Sir David King www.bis.gov.uk/foresight

JEBB S. 2011. Medical Research Council, Human Nutrition Research.
Cambridge, UK.

PENFIELD, W.,1975. Mystery of the Mind.: A Critical Study of
Consciousness and the   Human Brain. Princeton: Princeton University
Press. W.W.Norton & Co.

PROCHASKA, J, O, DiClemente, C,C, 1983. Stages and Processes of
Self-Change of Smoking: Toward an Integrative Model of Change. *J
Consult Clin Psychol 51 (3) 390-5.*

VANDENBROECK, P., Goossens, J., Clemens, M.,2007. Tackling
Obesity- Future Choices   – Building the Obesity System Map. London
: Foresight, Government Office, London.

CHAPTER 4

MAKING GOALS AND MEASURING SUCCESS

Chapter Objectives to:

- Clarify when it is appropriate to set goals

- How to best facilitate goal setting

Although this chapter is about goal setting clients are often not ready to set goals and the decision to change, of course remains with the client. Often interactions start with exploring the difficulties of making change. We have spent many sessions with clients exploring what their values are - their motivation. This intrinsic motivation is arguably the best rationale for change and not what *I* think should be the reason for change!

The Clients Own the Problem, Not you...

Constantly reminding ourselves that the client owns this problem, and subsequently the solution lies within that client, is essential for us to carry out interactions successfully. This helps us avoid jumping into solutions that the client has neither asked for is ready to undertake. This is a recurrent theme in counselling and effective 'helping'. Thomas Gordon in Parent Effectiveness Training shows how this remains true for helping small children and adults alike. Perhaps this is counter-intuitive as we have often learnt from an early age that correcting and informing are key roles and responsibilities in parenting. If so this no doubt impacts upon our adult interactions. We can clearly see where someone is going wrong and what the solution is!

Let's repeat that phrase *'we can clearly see where someone is going wrong and what the solution is'*

So we have problem + solution = advice (to correct)

The problem here is resistance/discord (disharmony or conflict), we listen to recordings of sessions made over the last few years and what we notice clearly is that nearly every time we offer unsolicited advice there is at least slight discord! No matter how gentle our advice in these sessions (and no matter how gentle the client's response to the nice nutritionist) there is still resistance either in the form of a statement that starts with 'yes but', or by the client diverting from the suggested advice and moving on to what is important to them.

As you are reading this, perhaps reflect how effective the strategy of advising is? You may feel it must be very effective, not effective at all, or sometimes effective. We ask our students how many of them have tried to 'advise' their mothers, boyfriends, girlfriends around diet and lifestyle - the response seems to show that many of them have. We then ask 'how was it?' Repeatedly the experience has been one of frustration even despair. In fact in years I have never seen a nodding head or indication that this has gone well/effectively despite classrooms full of people to ask the question to…

Yet people are concerned about their diet and lifestyle and often feel the need to change - how can this be?

Resistance

We propose that people really, really don't like being told what to do. There is, 'psychological-reactance' to suggestions foisted upon us. If we are told what we 'must do' we may even purposefully, wilfully head in the opposite direction. There are countless examples of this; one that stands out to me from Miller and Rollnick's (2002) text on motivational interviewing relates to 'Pinchgut Island' where sailors who drank were sent as a punishment, to an island where you would be chained without food or water and exposed to the elements. Not only that but flogging and ultimately hanging were punishments and yet people still drank…

Relate this to the smoker - who knows all about the ill-effects, potential risk of smoking, realistically how many people do not know of a connection between fatal disease and smoking? Yet they still smoke, the decision is not based upon knowing whether there is risk or not.

So the point about clients having ownership over the problem is not one made lightly- we really do need to invest ourselves of this idea - it is not our problem to fix yet we may be effective in facilitating the client to find their own solution.

Goal Setting

So when is the time to start goal setting? When the client suggests it would be a great start. I am not implying that we have no role in directing and strengthening the likelihood of talking about change, I am suggesting that if the client is not ready to start talking about change we should back off and follow them, listen to them, hear what they are saying and seek to understand better.

Goal setting is also clearly key to success. How often do we plan to lose weight, exercise more, eat less, save money stop drinking alcohol... The desire to change behaviour is present in most people.

A goal in the business coaching sense must be clear - i.e. '*I want to lose weight*' is not a clear goal but rather a general aspiration. Whereas '*I want to lose 5 kilograms by June the 30th*' is very clear, it presupposes action that would need to be taken between now and then - it is specific and measurable. In working with clients *when they decide* to set goals - we keep this firmly in mind.

In their excellent book on Health Behaviour Change Rollnick, Mason and Butler, (2010) discuss moving goals from the 'general to the specific'. An example they use is someone wishing to lose weight (i.e. very general) via strategy of eating less fatty food (more specific but still general) via not eating red meat during the week days (highly specific). This is the crux of effective goal setting whilst aspirations are unclear they may well remain as aspirations.

Gollwitzer talks about implementing intentions and the gap between aspiration and 'implementation' stating that intentions ('I want to join a gym in the new year') account for only 20-30% of actual behaviour. In short Gollwitzer's argument is that intention is only weakly correlated with actual behaviour. In motivational interviewing identifying, eliciting and strengthening change talk are key goals. Change talk relates to psycho-linguistics, i.e. the relationship between words people use and what they signify.

Perhaps when have a chat with a friend over coffee you have experienced this, the friend talks about what she 'really ought to do' and what she 'needs to do' when you compare this with the same friend talking about what she 'will do' and is 'going today tomorrow morning at 9.00 a.m.' the tone and the feeling of certainty you get is entirely different?

In motivational interviewing two levels of 'change talk' are talked about, they are either: *preparatory* or *mobilising* language (Miller and Rollnick, 2012). Desire, Ability, Reason and need are defined as *preparatory* language whereas commitment and taking steps are *mobilising* language. In essence the mobilising language is stronger this is something you know of course, every time you chat to a friend over coffee and he says something like: '*I really should do some exercise*' (preparatory) versus '*I am going to join the gym in the morning*' (mobilising) you gain a sense of which of these statements is most likely to lead to action!

D esire

A ability **Preparatory language (e.g. 'I should')**

R eason

N eed

C ommitment **Mobilising Language (e.g. 'I will')**

T aking steps

So in terms of implementing intentions - a person is more likely to make change when they are using mobilising language rather than preparatory language. The preparatory may or may not be prelude to change, as in the example above 'I *should* do some exercise' is weak compared to '*I am going to*'. Motivational interviewing seeks to elicit and strengthen change talk. You can see how the words above represent the likelihood of change taking place. Going back to the chatting to a friend over coffee analogy - think about this the next time you are talking to someone about change. Are they using preparatory or mobilising language?

Dave Rosengren's book on developing Motivational interviewing skills offers excellent exercises for identifying and strengthening change talk. We also propose Motivational Interviewing training/workshops delivered by a motivational interviewing network of trainers, trainer as an excellent adjunct to your weight-management practice MINT.

In coaching the GROW process (Griffiths & Kaday 2004) is often used, which relates to Goal, Reality, Obstacles and Options and Way forward. Again there is the idea that a **goal** must be clear e.g. 5 kilos weight loss by June 30th, but also that the **reality** must be stated i.e.: '*where am I now in relation to this behaviour change?*' I could be not exercising regularly yet, or really controlling what I eat in any systematic manner, so this is stating the reality in the same terms as the goal. The **Obstacles** - these could be reticence to join a fitness club or begin walking to work because I have no comfortable shoes or I am worried about wasting money. Options might be to explore gym membership and different rates/costs associated with this and to investigate a new pair of walking shoes. Finally one of these options might be a **way forward**, e.g. I choose to visit a shoe shop at lunchtime on Monday to look at shoes.

Frustrations avoided by motivational interviewing

A frustration in our experience is counsellors wanting to get a change out of everyone from every interaction! This might be implausible. Heaping change upon change in someone who needs to move slowly in order to sustain change is not going to help.

In Motivational Interviewing the process often starts with exploring client's motivation and confidence to change:

Ascertain: Motivation

> *'What is it that you feel you would achieve by losing this weight?'*

Importance

> *'You spoke about wanting to lose weight - on a scale of 1 to 10 with 10 being very important indeed and 1 being not important at all - how important is this for you right now?'*

OR

> *'You identified making changes to your diet and taking more exercise as the key elements to successfully bringing your weight down. I wonder how confident, on a scale of 1 to 10 (with 1 representing not at all and 10 representing very) you feel about making these changes?'*

The use of these scaling questions is that there is opportunity to explore the issue further for example when a client says in response to the scaling question: 'I am a 3' we can choose to explore further with: *'how come you are not a zero?'*

'Well I have started to do this before...' i.e. the client is inclined to talk about positive reasons for change - rather than saying *'why are you only a three and not a...'* which may well incite the client to start listing all the negative reasons for not changing.

With scaling questions, however low the response, with the exception of zero, there is always the opportunity to say 'why not zero?'

When this has been explored we might try:

'OK so there are some reasons to give you confidence (list these back to the client) now tell me what would move you form a 3 to a five'

Anchoring

The issue of 'anchoring' a goal is important for Small Changes. We are most especially concerned that the client has (for themselves not us) a clear picture of what they are going to do, how they will achieve this and when. I include an extract below which examples both goal setting and anchoring the goal.

Further work by Gollwitzer and Brandstatter, emphasises how powerful this can be. In an experiment that supposedly tried to identify how people spent their holiday time. Researchers asked two groups to write a report on how they had spent Christmas eve and this was to be produced no more than 48 hours after the event. In one group implementation intentions were formed by indicating exactly where and when they intended to write the report in the other group were not requested to pick a time or place. The implementation intentions group returned three quarters of the questionnaires the other group returned a third.

Case-study: Anchoring

SC: *'you mentioned starting to run again - is that what you'd like to do?'*

C: *'I think it's the best option, I mean I've done it before I enjoyed it I just need to start again'*

SC: *'is there anything stopping you?'*

C: *'I don't think so, the only thing stopping me is getting started...'*

SC: *'it's difficult to motivate yourself?'*

pauses

C: *'if I started then that would be it I'd go all the time it's more the first attempt getting my shorts and trainers on and going out'*

SC: *'so you'd like to run again and you've done it before how often did you run?'*

C: *'half an hour forty minutes each night'*

SC: *'and now you'd like to do the same?*

C: *'yes I'll run every night once I've started'*

SC: *'you don't run at all at the moment?'*

C: *'it's been ohh 18 months or two years'*

SC: *'would you run every night right from the start?*

C: *'I'd probably build up to it, I might be a bit sore at first - so I might try three times a week'*

SC: *'do you want to set a goal for this and we'll catch up on it next week?'*

C: *'why not, let's go for it'*

SC: *'so you say three times a week to begin with but what if for your small change you got those trainers and shorts out and did one easy jog to meet your commitment and if you do more than that it's a bonus'*

The above (real) example is a large change in fact. Many Small Change goals are much more modest than beginning to run, but the goal must match the client. In this case someone who had run fairly recently (i.e. months/2 years ago rather than decades) and had the confidence that they could do it, is very different to someone with no or no recent history of being physically active. Often clients are choosing to drink a glass a water each day - this is fairly common at the first session. This of course offers the scope to exceed the goal and then feel greatly affirmed at the follow-up session.

Another issue which we have frequently discussed, is the fact that every interaction with a client has some goal, in the sense of a meaningful conversation. That goal may seem abstract if we go into the interaction thinking of change in terms of always relating to uptake of exercise and change to diet. We might, however, consider that a decision to think about something represents change. So clients may decide to think through their motivation, or reasons for change, in their own time, or to explore other reasons for their behaviour. This could be much more important and effective than pushing for change - trying to make each interaction goal orientated in terms of actually changing behaviour.

We like to reflect in my own sessions thus:

'Who owns this problem?'

'What am I trying to do in this consultation?'

We are able to carry out this reflection as very often we have permission from clients to record our sessions so we can play them back and listen to them under supervision. This may seem onerous, but we cannot think of another way of being able to continually reflect and analyse practice so that we make it better.

Table 1. Is the client's goal clear?

Goal (general)	How will you do that? (more specific but still general)	What sort of exercise, where when, how will this be achieved? (very specific)	Is this likely, achievable/realistic?
Lose weight	Exercise more and eat less fatty food	No treat foods mon-fri, circuit training class mon and Fri	

Assessment Questions

1. Goal setting is essential to every interaction and we must motivate the client to make change T or F

2. Confidence rulers allow the opportunity to further explore the positive reasons, which underpin the likelihood of a client being successful. T or F

3. GROW, is a process that suggests goals must be clear rather than vague aspirations T or F

4. Goal setting is decided by the client and not the facilitator, when the client is not ready to change or 'action plan' it is better for us to leave the door open and have the client return later than to push on for problem resolution T or F

5. The stated intention to carry out a behaviour never predicts whether it will happen or not… T or F

Answers in Appendix 1

References

GRIFFITHS, B and Kaday, C (2004) *Grow your Own Carrot Motivate Yourself to Success!* Lighten source Milton Keynes

BRECKON, J. JOHNSON, L.H. and HUTCHISON, A. (2008). Physical Activity Counseling Content and Competency: A Systematic Review. *Journal of Physical Activity and Health,* **5,** 398-417.

GOLLWITZER, P.M (1999) Implementation Intention, American Psychologist 54, (7) 493-503,

GOLLWITZER, P.M. Brandstatter, V (1997) Implementation intentions and effective goal pursuit. Journal of Personality and Social Psychology, 73, 186-199

ROLLNICK, S, Mason, P and Butler, C (2010) *Health behaviour Change A Guide For Counsellors* Churchill Livingstone

ROSENGREN, D (2009) Building Motivational Interviewing Skills a counsellor workbook Guildford Press Lond

CHAPTER 5

FOOD: HELEN BERRY

Chapter Objectives to:

- Explore the physiological predispositions to obesity and weight gain.

- Understand how aspects of diet contribute to weight gain and associated poor health.

- Explore environmental factors which contribute to obesity.

Amount and type

Current emphasis in the UK is on obesity as a result of lifestyle choice, the responsibility of the individual rather than a public health issue. This makes it harder, though not impossible, to use the law to fight rising obesity levels. Food is more difficult to legislate for in health terms than smoking or drinking, because it is unavoidable. Smokers have the option to give up smoking and alcoholics to give up drinking, but we all have to eat. A wide evidence base is needed to determine the contribution to obesity of factors such as geography, climate, economics, media, culture and patterns of food trade and distribution, before effective laws can be made.

The problem is not so much food itself as the type and amount of food we eat. Recent research has shown that people using larger forks eat less, possibly because the bigger forks fool their brains into thinking they've eaten more than they have. The brain responds to external cues such as the amount of food left on your plate when prompting you to feel full. If using a bigger fork makes more visible inroads into the contents of your plate this may help with the time lag between actual fullness and the recognition of that feeling by the brain. So far, however, these results only seem to apply to big servings on large plates.

A couple of other tried and trusted strategies are to eat slowly and use smaller plates. It takes about 15 to 20 minutes for your brain to pick up satiety signals, and it's been shown many times that people given larger plates will eat more.

Another way of cutting down the amount you eat is to repeat the same meals, for example by sticking to the same healthy breakfast or lunch every day. This is known as habituation. The more frequently you expose someone to a stimulus, whether that stimulus is food, or something else like a loud noise, the weaker their reaction becomes. A new stimulus, such as the arrival of pudding, often results in the recovery of appetite, even though the person had just been feeling quite full and did not need any more calories. Conversely, if the extra temptations are not there and you know exactly what to expect, you are unlikely to overeat.

Good food/bad food?

It could be argued that much of the so-called food we buy is in fact a chemically derived approximation of food designed to make more money for food manufacturers. Manufacturers and retailers would say that no food is bad as such; its effects on health depend on how much is eaten and how often and that is up to the individual. After all, no one is forcing you to eat too much chocolate, cheese, chips or cake.

This may be true, strictly speaking, but it's a very disingenuous argument. People who lead very full, stressful lives are persuaded by marketing and advertising ploys that certain products will keep them and their families happy, save time, effort and money and even make them feel healthy and virtuous because of the reduced fat/added vitamins etc. Many companies now have 'healthy food' ranges, but these vary widely in nutrient value and content and are promoted instead of natural, minimally processed foods.

Activity

We are often told that we eat far less than our prehistoric ancestors and yet we are still putting on weight. This is partly because our technology-filled lives mean we use far less energy on a daily basis. Many people go to the gym or dance classes or jogging for a couple of hours two or three times a week, think they eat reasonably well and can't understand why the weight isn't shifting. It doesn't occur to them to consider the drive to and from work or anywhere else more than a couple of minutes' walk away, the desk job where they communicate by phone and email instead of going a few yards down the office to talk to someone, the evening sat in front of the TV.

There is evidence to show that short bursts of activity throughout the day do far more to boost people's metabolism and use up calories than two or three longer sessions spread through the week. At the same time it may be that many people actually aren't eating enough because of worries about their weight, and what they are eating is not of sufficiently good quality. Their bodies are making them crave more food in an attempt to get the nutrients they are being deprived of, but lack of knowledge and years of eating poor quality food mean people are more likely to meet this craving with high fat and high sugar foods than those which would do them more good.

Eating and the brain/attitudes

At its most basic, eating is a means of conveying energy into the body as part of the cerebral supply chain. Comfort eating, or increased intake of calorie-dense foods, may provide some people with extra glucose needed by the brain in times of stress, helping to stabilise mood. Obesity may result when the brain is unable to demand and receive glucose from the body efficiently. This is known as inefficient brain pull and results in some of the increased energy intake being stored in fat and muscle tissue before it gets to the brain.

People with inefficient brain pull tend to have low sympatho-adrenal activity or faulty stress systems and evidence shows this is a predictor of weight gain. This may be due to adaptation to chronic stress; depression and anxiety have also been linked and children whose mothers experienced traumatic or stressful events in pregnancy had high blood sugar in adulthood and were more likely to gain weight.

It's hard to believe that there are many people who haven't got at least some awareness of the government's healthy eating messages. Large numbers of people are on diets at any one time; clearly many of us are greatly concerned about our weight and our children's weight and the effect it has on our health, appearance and self-esteem. We want to know how to make it work, permanently, without making ourselves and everyone around us miserable. We forget that we aren't machines; our nutritional needs vary and we also have cultural and social needs which are partly met by the preparation and sharing of food.

Many people will know the constant cycle of working hard to get the winter weight off in time for the summer, the sense of achievement and then the gradual loss of motivation to keep the new svelte figure as winter approaches again with all its temptations. There's a constant feeling of guilt and failure, of being weak-willed, and a frustration with the seeming inevitability of repeating the same pattern over and over without apparently learning from experience, but maybe this cycle is perfectly natural.

Humans and other mammals are programmed to store fat to see them through times when food is scarce. The increased availability of ripe fruits with their high fructose content in the autumn provides an energy source which not only meets immediate needs, but may also help to raise fat stores for the winter. Shortage of food in winter and in other circumstances may not be a problem for many of us now, but a fluctuation of a few pounds through the year is not a calamity as long as weight stays within a healthy range. This range might be easier to maintain if our attitude to food was more balanced and concerned with long-term health and wellbeing, rather than obsessive and focussed on short-term goals.

Eating and taste

Fat increases the palatability of foods, making them more enjoyable and rewarding. Overeating and obesity are related to a greater than normal sense of reward from food which overrides the body's natural satiety signals. Special receptors in the mouth and small intestine should react with fat to help regulate how much is absorbed, but this system seems to be overpowered by a high fat diet. Reduced ability to detect fatty acids in the mouth has been linked with higher intakes of fat and total calories and higher BMI. The gut signals the brain, by mechanisms not yet fully understood, to regulate gastrointestinal function and food intake when prompted by sensing nutrients, especially fatty acids, in the small intestine.

Rodent studies also show that taste and smell vary between individuals. Taste is linked to other behaviours such as the regulation of food and liquid intake. The ingestion of food is probably determined by several genes, many of which are yet to be discovered. Sweetness sensitivity is known to vary in humans - in other words some people really do have a sweeter tooth than others.

Past eating patterns

It's simplistic to talk of a 'Stone Age Diet' since evidence shows that early *homo sapiens* varied their diet as least as much as we do today depending on their environment and circumstances, but it's interesting to compare some basic information on eating patterns given that we are physiologically more or less the same.

Total calorie intake for Palaeolithic man was between 2 and 7 times as high as ours, but their food was bulkier, more fibrous and less calorie-dense, which suggests the greater part of their days were spent on the move looking for food. They ate twice as much fruit and vegetables, but less carbohydrate in total, as they had very little cereal or refined carbohydrate and added sugars. Protein intake was higher, but there was no dairy apart from mother's milk. Fat intake was similar in amount to ours, but contained more polyunsaturated and essential fatty acids; interestingly, cholesterol intake was higher. They drank more water and generally their diet was alkaline and potassium-rich, whereas ours is acidic and high in sodium.

Levels of micronutrients were higher, for example they had 4 times as much vitamin D from being outside all day. Humans lost the ability to synthesise vitamin C in the late Eocene period (about 56 million years ago). This coincided with global cooling, which could have reduced the availability of fruit; vitamin C partially blocks the effects of fructose and as fruit ripens, fructose content increases and vitamin C falls, so that fruit is most likely to cause weight gain just before winter when fat stores are needed. This was a period of numerous mammal extinctions and this mutation may have been essential to human survival.

Conversely the ready availability of fruits such as berries in summer with their high vitamin C content, more water and less sugar would help to block the fat storage effects of fructose at a time when it was important to be lean and fit for hunting and gathering and taking care of your companions.

Evidence from northern Kenya shows that where food was easily available early humans were foragers with a varied diet, eating whatever came to hand, including small land and water-living animals. They lived in a variety of habitats and ate a wide range of foods using a combination of hunting, foraging and scavenging. Plant and animal/fish consumption seems to have been about equal, at least in East Africa.

Migration and cultural adaptations may have led to nutritional changes that genetic evolution couldn't keep up with, leading to the development of diseases and conditions such as obesity, heart disease and various cancers. For instance, early Inuit remains show evidence of osteoporosis due to lack of plant food; high intake of animal protein raises the acidity of the body environment and thus the risk of osteoporosis. Modern humans who still lead a Stone Age lifestyle have very low rates of degenerative disease. It may also be true that early humans didn't live as long as us and therefore may not have had time to develop some of the degenerative diseases we suffer from.

Problems with dietary changes

Today protein intake in the west has fallen for several decades, but consumption of added sugars has risen dramatically from 4lbs a year per person in 1700 to an average of 150lbs today. Studies of modern Australian Aborigines suggest that insulin resistance may have developed as a survival mechanism when eating a diet high in protein and low in carbohydrate and fat. This causes problems when the diet is switched to one high in fat and refined carbohydrate, but switching back again at least partially reverses the ill effects.

Loss of bone mass

Weight loss due to calorie restriction and yo-yo dieting is often accompanied by loss of bone mass. A weight loss diet for both men and women with around 108 grams of protein daily has been found to preserve bone mineral better than one with around 70 grams. A study of obese women showed that those who lost weight after bariatric surgery also lost significant amounts of bone mass, possibly partly due to the rapid speed of weight loss. Hormonal factors, such as Insulin-like Growth Factor 1 (IGF-1), are associated with this process. IGF-1levels were significantly lower in those who had bariatric surgery compared with those who did not. Exercise may offset these adverse effects, but the research on this is inconclusive.

What is well established is that maintaining adequate bone strength and density depends on having adequate muscle mass, which means eating enough high-quality protein. Dietary protein may be as vital to bone health as calcium and vitamin D. The nutrient deficiencies, decreased hormone production and decrease in physical activity which accompany the usual ageing process, may also cause loss of muscle tissue. At present little attention is paid to making sure that elderly fracture patients get enough protein and calcium.

Despite a widely held belief that high-protein diets (especially animal protein) result in bone resorption and increased urinary calcium, higher protein diets are actually associated with greater bone mass and fewer fractures, provided calcium intake is adequate. Increasing the intake of alkalinizing fruits and vegetables might be more useful and beneficial than reducing protein intake.

Types of food provision

Wild plant and animal foods were staples of hunter-gatherer societies and are still actively managed by many communities around the world today, but these foods are not included in official figures for values of natural resources in spite of the huge contribution they make. When food security tends to concentrate on cultivated foods there's a danger of forgetting to protect the ecosystems which provide wild foods. Agricultural expansion reduces wild ecosystems and threatens wild species.

The traditional view of humans progressing from savage hunters to civilised agrarians through to industrialisation is now challenged as inaccurate. The current argument is that methods of finding food simply vary with the local environment and different methods often coexist. Many societies, while not farming animals in a way we would recognise, develop a symbiotic relationship with local wildlife which is a sort of pre-farming. There is a continuum from completely 'wild' to completely 'domesticated' rather than a clear division between the two, which necessitates a closer awareness of and involvement with the natural environment than most of us in the West have today.

Biodiversity is lost when land is homogenised for intensive agriculture and mono-systems of crop growing. Cultivated wheat, corn and rice provide more than half the world's daily calorie and protein requirements and just 12 cultivated species make up 80% of dietary intake. Conversely, there are many communities that use wild animals and plants in the hundreds, with a much greater dietary diversity, where there is no such thing as a weed since plants have multiple uses beyond food alone.

Wild foods tend to have low energy density and be good sources of micronutrients and these attributes vary to suit the time of year and likely needs of the consumer. They are usually superior in nutritional content to shop-bought foods; where communities have moved away from their traditional diets to modern Western diets there has been a rapid and very noticeable negative impact on nutritional status.

Phytochemicals in plants are a major part of their immune systems, helping to protect against pests, pathogens and pollution as well as other stressors such as weather conditions and poor soil. Some of these have developed to help plants adapt to their environment as they are unable to escape it; for instance they often have a natural resilience to weather changes, which is absent or undeveloped in cultivated species, or they may develop a bitter taste to protect them from being eaten. Many of these phytochemicals have a positive effect on human health, which we are only just beginning to understand.

Diet and health

The sequencing of the human genome means we can now study how diet effects health on an individual basis. Diet should be a key component of preventative health strategy but health budgets tend to concentrate on treatment rather than prevention. In the industrialised world food is abundant, but restricted in terms of nutritional content compared with Palaeolithic-type diets. In the developing world a scarcity of food often leads to under-nutrition, but health problems also arise because of the introduction of western-style diets for those who can afford them. A list of 12 factors for poor health and life expectancy around the world (not just the developing world) published in a 2002 WHO report included 8 nutritional ones, namely:

Underweight in children and mothers, iron deficiency, zinc deficiency, vitamin A deficiency, obesity, high cholesterol, high blood pressure and alcohol.

Food taboos

Food taboos are common and widespread and have been around for a long time. Sometimes they seem sensible and logical, with a sound scientific basis. For example, Jewish dietary laws stipulate that utensils used in connection with foods which contain meat must always be kept separate from those used for other foods; a wise precaution to avoid cross-contamination. Often, food taboos have a religious origin; they are associated with holy days and festivals and intended to set believers apart from non-believers, but also designed to protect and promote the health of the faithful.

Rites of passage such as the onset of menstruation, pregnancy, childbirth, lactation, and events like hunting, fighting, weddings and funerals are frequently accompanied by certain rules regarding food. In certain tribes of West Malaysia, pregnant women are supposed only to eat small animals with weak spirits, and after childbirth to eat gruel for a week and then to eat alone for 6 weeks.

Food resources can be protected or used more efficiently by applying taboos. A form of rationing can be applied to prevent a resource being used up by restricting its consumption to certain groups of people. Food taboos can also be used to emphasise and underline differences in status, with women and children often allowed less nutritional variety than men. This can lead to essential nutrients for these groups being limited, and the restrictions imposed are not always strictly adhered to, showing that there can be some degree of leeway in certain circumstances.

On the other hand there are many food taboos which make no sense at all to outsiders and whose origins are lost in the mists of time, or based on superstition. What is beyond the pale for one group can be quite normal for another. Perhaps the most important purpose of food taboos is to reinforce a sense of belonging to a particular group and having a distinct identity apart from other groups.

Food taboos exist in all countries and cultures. As well as pertaining to particular groups they can also be very individual and personal, so it is very important to take this into account when trying to change people's eating habits.

Food myths

These are beliefs learned from family and friends, gleaned from the popular press or perhaps hangovers from past scientific understanding which has been superseded by more up to date knowledge, which can hamper attempts to lose weight and keep it off. The following are examples that can be expanded with reference to relevant studies.

Detox diets are a good way to start weight loss.

Your liver, kidneys, intestines, lungs and skin are designed to get rid of waste matter and toxins. They do it every day very efficiently and you can help the process and keep everything in good working order by getting regular exercise and eating a balanced, healthy diet most of the time. So-called detox diets can leave you tired and short of essential nutrients and money.

Butter versus margarine

Butter is a natural product, which people in the northern hemisphere have adapted to over thousands of years. It contains vitamins A, D, E and K and small amounts of B vitamins as well as calcium and other minerals. Butter is well known for its high saturated fat content, which has been linked to raised LDL cholesterol levels but it also contains mono and polyunsaturated fats. Many people find the taste superior to that of margarine. In this country we like it salted and because of that and the saturated fat, it's probably best to limit consumption, but that doesn't mean going without unless you already have high blood cholesterol levels, or a family history of them.

Most margarine now, especially for spreading rather than cooking, no longer contains dangerous trans fats. Full fat margarine and butter contain about the same calories, but lower fat margarines are readily available. Margarine is low in saturated fat and has vitamins and minerals added. Which you use is really a matter of personal preference, but in either case keep the amounts sparing.

Dairy is fattening

It can be, but there are plenty of low fat options available, or if you really don't like these, eat smaller amounts of the full fat versions and experiment with reducing fat levels gradually, perhaps mixing full and low fat products.

Low fat is always best

We need some fat so that we can process fat-soluble vitamins and for various other vital functions. Processed low fat foods often replace the taste and texture lost through removing fat with added sugar and fillers so always check the labels. It's also perfectly possible to make your own low fat versions of many of your favourite foods without spending money on ready meals.

Nuts are fattening

Nuts are high in healthy unsaturated fats and contain fibre, vitamins and minerals. They are a good source of protein for vegetarians. However they are a very concentrated source of nutrients and calories and should therefore be eaten in small amounts.

Eggs raise cholesterol

Studies have shown that most people can eat as many eggs as they want unless they have an innate tendency to high cholesterol levels. Generally only about a third of our cholesterol comes from what we eat and the rest is made by the body.

Salads are a healthy option

They are if made with a variety of good quality fresh ingredients and not smothered in fatty sauces and dressings. Keep added extras like cheese, croutons, and processed meats to a minimum and don't use dressings, or serve them separately so you can control how much you add.

Fresh is always best

Not if it's spent several weeks in transit or storage followed by several more days hanging about in your kitchen. Frozen fruit and vegetables retain higher levels of vitamins for longer and even canned produce can have useful levels of minerals, fibre and some vitamins. Both can be stored for a considerable time without effecting their nutritional value.

Raw vegetables are best

Overcooking kills vitamin C, but some light cooking is needed to break down the cell walls of vegetables like carrots so that the nutrients are more easily available to the body. another positive e.g. of cooking is the availability of lycopene in tomatoes which are cooked rather than raw - so raw is not always best.

Some food uses more calories to digest than it contains

No. Some foods are just very low-calorie. While they may be good healthy options as part of a balanced diet, regimes which rely almost totally on one or two of these foods, such as the grapefruit or cabbage soup diets, work temporarily because of the drastic reduction in calorie intake, but are unsustainable and nutritionally inadequate.

Carbohydrates are bad

Simple carbohydrates are digested and broken down to glucose very quickly. If the glucose isn't used by the body straight away it will be stored as fat for future use. Complex carbohydrates release energy slowly and steadily and come as a package with fibre and a range of micronutrients. Go for minimally processed wholefoods most of the time and save the sweets and shop-bought cakes and biscuits for an occasional treat.

You shouldn't eat after 5 or 6pm

There is some evidence which suggests that we process food differently at different times of day, but generally eating at night effects your weight because you are taking in extra calories. If you normally start eating later in the day and you eat sensibly and don't consume more calories than you use, eating at night should not be a major problem. If you feel it makes a difference in your case, then look at changing your eating patterns.

I can't help being overweight, it's my genes

There may be something in this, but most of the problem will almost certainly be the result of environment and bad habits. If you know being fat runs in the family use that knowledge to help establish good eating habits and avoid falling into bad ones.

My weight gain is due to a food intolerance

Probably not! This is quite rare, but if you suspect it ask your doctor to arrange tests. Don't self-diagnose or waste money on quack 'therapists'. If you have a genuine problem you will need proper advice and treatment. Cutting out any food or food group will lead to weight loss because you are cutting calories, but doing so without the right information could mean missing out on essential nutrients and jeopardizing your health.

Assessment Questions:

1. Low sympatho-adrenal activity associated with inefficient brain pull is a predictor of weight gain. T or F?

2. Humans are programmed to store fat to see them through times when food is scarce. T or F?

3. What has been linked with a reduced ability to detect fatty acids in the mouth?

4. Are detox diets a good idea?

5. The Palaeolithic diet was acidic and high in sodium. T or F?

6. Adequate protein intake is needed to maintain bone mass. T or F?

Answers in Appendix 1:

BIBLIOGRAPHY

BARUCHA, Z. and PRETTY, J. (2010). The roles and values of wild foods in agricultural systems. [online]. *Philosophical transactions of the Royal Society B Biological Sciences,* **365** (1554), 2913-2926.

BOUGHTER, J. D. and BACHMANOV, A. A. (2007). Behavioural genetics and taste. [online]. *BMC Neuroscience,* **8** (53).

BOYD-EATON, S., KONNER, M. J. and CORDAIN, L. (2010). Diet-dependent acid load, Palaeolithic nutrition, and evolutionary health promotion. [online]. *American Journal of Clinical Nutrition,* **91** (2) 295-297.

CASAGRANDE, D.S. et al. (2010). Bone Mineral Density and Nutritional Profile in Morbidly Obese Women. [online]. *Obesity Surgery,* **20**:1372–1379.

EPSTEIN, L. H. et al. (2009). Habituation as a determinant of human food intake. [online]. *Psychological Review,* **116** (2), 384-487.

FAIRWEATHER-TAIT, S. J. (2003). Human nutrition and food research: opportunities and challenges in the post-genomic era. [online]. *Philosophical transactions of the Royal Society B Biological Sciences,* **358** (1438), 1709-1727.

HEANEY, R. P. AND LAYMAN, D. K. (2008). Amount and type of protein influences bone health. [online]. *American Journal of Clinical Nutrition,* **87** (5), 1567S-1570S.

IRITI, M. and FAORO, F. (2009). Chemical diversity and defence metabolism: how plants cope with pathogens and ozone pollution. [online]. *International Journal of Molecular Sciences,* **10** (8), 3371-3399.

JOHNSON, R. J. et al. (2010). Theodore E. Woodward Award – The Evolution of Obesity: Insights from the Mid-Miocene. [online]. *Transactions of the American Clinical and Climatological Association*, **121**, 295-308.

LITTLE, T.J. AND FEINLE-BISSET, C. (2010). Oral and Gastrointestinal Sensing of Dietary Fat and Appetite Regulation in Humans: Modification by Diet and Obesity. [online]. *Frontiers in Neuroscience*, **4** (178), 1-9.

MARTIN, R. (2008). The role of law in the control of obesity in England: looking at the contribution of low to a healthy food culture. [online]. *Australia and New Zealand Health Policy*, **5** (21).

MEYER-ROCHOW, V. B. (2009). Food Taboos: their origins and purposes. [online]. *Journal of Ethnobiology and Ethnomedicine.* **5** (18).

MISHRA, A., MISHRA, H. and MASTERS, T. M. (2011). The Influence of Bite Size on Quantity of Food Consumed: A Field Study. [online]. *Journal of Consumer Research*, **38**. DOI: 10.1086/660838.

DE PASCUAL-TERESA, S., MORENA, D. A. and GARCIA-VIGUERA, C.C. (2010). Flavonols and anthocyanins in cardiovascular health: a review of current evidence. [online]. *International Journal of Molecular Sciences,* **11** (4), 1679-1703.

PETERS, A. and LANGEMANN, D. (2010). Stress and eating behaviour. [online]. *F1000 Biology Reports,* **2** (13).

ROLLS, E. T. (2010). Taste, olfactory and food texture reward processing in the brain and obesity. [online]. *International Journal of Obesity (London).*

STEELE, T. E. (2010). A unique hominin menu dated to 1.95 million years ago. [online]. *Proceedings of the National Academy of Sciences of the United States of America,* **107** (24), 10771-10772.

STROHLE, A., HAHN, A. and SEBASTIAN, A. (2010). Estimation of the diet-dependent net acid load in 229 worldwide historically studied hunter-gatherer societies. [online]. *American Journal of Clinical Nutrition,* **91** (2), 406-412.

CHAPTER 6

PHYSICAL ACTIVITY

Chapter objectives to:

- Clarify the 'guidelines' for physical activity

- Give key examples of how awareness can be raised around physical activity levels in your client/self

- Clarify the fact that these guidelines count for nothing! (if the client didn't ask for them...)

Physical activity levels in the UK

Ever since Jeremy Morris completed seminal studies on bus drivers and conductors (Morris & Campbell 1958), postmen and others in the 1950's, the relationship between physical activity and heart disease has become clearer. Morris found that the drivers suffered more heart attacks than the conductors and that the protective factor for the conductors was being on their feet and moving more...

Physical activity levels are low in the UK and U.S alike. Health Survey for England data showed that, in 2003, only 37% of men and 24% of women met the current physical activity guidelines suggested by the Government. In 2003 over one third of English adults were inactive, that is, participated in less than one occasion of 30 minutes activity a week.

This of course has implications for the country's disease profile and in particular the levels of coronary heart disease, cardiovascular disease and type 2 diabetes. Effective insulin sensitivity, a working circulatory system and efficient cardiac functioning all appear to be promoted by moving around more. A difficulty may then be in being more specific about which types and intensities of exercise confer benefit. The epidemiology around exercise (for e.g's see bibliography: Morris, Blair and Connelly, Hardman, Pafenbarger) has shown the protective relationship of PA on health. In exercise prescription the recommendation gets detailed with information suggesting a combination of moderate intensity aerobic exercise (walking, cycling, swimming, gardening: at a rate that leaves you feeling warmer and breathing harder but still able to converse) and resistance training (weights or machines or push-up, sit-up type exercise) twice a week. Adopting this kind of exercise a mixture of both aerobic and anaerobic seems to be the most potent enhancer of insulin sensitivity McArdle Katch and Katch (2007).

Good news on physical activity

The great news about physical activity and the reason why in public health terms it can be described as 'best buy', is that it works at relatively low levels of participation to improve health chances and lower risk indices. The government's 30 minutes a day of moderate intensity exercise on most or all days of the week is a case in point. This represents half an hour's brisk walking a day! A commonly quoted statistic is that this level of participation will reduce the chances of a (previously sedentary) person developing coronary heart disease. Further to this the Harvard Alumni study showed that by far the greatest benefits were to be had by moving from being sedentary (not active at all) to being moderately active as per the government guidelines just mentioned.

In the study it was also noted that life expectancy steadily increases in individuals completing physical activity ranging from 500Kcal to 3500Kcal per week (a value of 6-8 hours of strenuous exercise) McArdle Katch and Katch p.906 (2007)

In this study no further health or longevity benefits were conferred by doing more than 3500Kcal worth of exercise.

It is important to note that being active at a younger age does seemingly nothing for protecting your health in older age - it is lifelong physical activity and responses that relate to your recent physical activity that are important. It is also perhaps interesting to examine the relationship between exercise and all-cause mortality (all causes of death). In the Harvard Alumni study it was noted that regular exercise countered the effects of:

- *Excess bodyweight*
- *Smoking*
- *Genetic tendency toward early death*
- *Hypertension*

That is to say *despite* the presence of the above factors in any of the 17,000 people involved in the study, exercise exerted an independent protective effect against death. Tremendous benefit has been gained in terms of understanding the nature and extent of physical activities protective effect on health through the work of Morris, Paffenbarger, Blair, Connelly and Hardman.

To add to all this evidence the World Health Organisation's world health report also suggests that 3% of all disease burden in industrialised nations is due to inactivity.

'Choosing Activity' is the exercise section of the Government white paper Choosing Health. The targets set out in this paper include increasing adult participation in at least 30 minutes moderate activity on at least five days of the week to 30%. Given the above statement regarding men and women's current participation levels this involves doubling the uptake in the fifteen years following publication i.e. 2005-2020. This is where you come in! This book is likely to be published in late 2007/early 2008 that gives us all eight years or so to help out…

Age related physical activity statistics

If you take the *'Choosing Activity'* and the BHF's excellent statistics site as starting points to understand some of the problems facing you in physical activity promotion you will see that rates of participation decline with age. At 16-24 years of age 53% of men and 30% of women met the activity guidelines, but at 25-34 this reduces to 44% and 29% respectively and then between 35-44 men drop again to 41% and women go up to 30%. So there appears to be a relationship between sex, age and participation in physical activity. If we look towards the older age groups you may immediately surmise that at ages of 65 and above immobility and problems such as osteoporosis are more prevalent and therefore this explains lower activity levels. Physiology studies on longevity decrepitude, exercise and protection from disease tend to show that although there is an accepted decrease in functional capacity *(for instance muscular atrophy where studies clearly show a reduced cross sectional area size in muscles particularly noticeable as people move into their 50's and 60's)* there is also considerable gain to be made by people of both sexes in their seventies from resistance and aerobic training. So what is it that happens to the people in the younger groups? Do the 16-24 year old males play sport and then give up at 25? Do the 45year old women get worried at 35 and start to do more?

The female statistics show remarkable consistency from 16-54 with levels remaining almost the same. Although these questions remain unanswered one thing that appears evident is that people of different ages and sexes participate at different levels – this may create an argument for targeting interventions at specific groups. Moreover as we shall discuss in behavioural change interventions should probably be targeted at the individual and involve them in the planning.

Look at the table overleaf to see the relationship between sex, age and participation in (higher than the minimum suggested prescription for) physical activity.

Information adapted from the British Heart Foundation statistics website:

Phys act > than minimum reccs *	Age 16-24	25-34	35-44	45-54	55-64	65-74	75 & over	Mean
Male	53%	44%	41%	38%	32%	17%	8%	37%
Female	30%	29%	30%	31%	23%	13%	3%	24%

* 30 mins moderate intensity walking on most days of the week

Walking recommendation:

10,000 steps a day and the exercise prescription of 30 minutes 'moderate' (e.g. brisk walking - feeling warmer, heart rate increased, breathing rate increased but still able to carry on a conversation) exercise on most days of the week.

We need to be careful not to confuse the above message with the message for people who are, or have been obese, the 30 minute brisk walking message is different in that it applies to all people for protection of health. The Department of Health recommend that people who are trying to lose weight, or maintain weight loss already achieved, should aim for sixty to ninety minutes a day of activity. These findings are confirmed by Department of Health and research carried out in the United States Jakicic (2008) and confirmed by the habits of people successful at weight loss as studied by Klem et al. (1997).

Clarify the fact that these guidelines count for nothing! *(if the client didn't ask for them...)*

NB although guidelines can be very useful to people seeking advice - we are suggesting they should be given out cautiously and within the framework of the Small Changes approach *when they are asked for or permission is obtained.* What is meant by this last statement is that when a client suggests they are confused by what or how much they are supposed to do it may be pertinent to then say:

'would it help here if I explained the guidelines for people wanting to lose weight?'

The effect this has is dramatic in terms of clients being receptive to information.

Participants, of course, often have very low levels of physical activity and *any* increase in levels may be positive. Our goal is to encourage any increase in energy expenditure rather than meeting government targets. So if, for instance, a client walks ten minutes a day instead of five minutes this represents a 100% increase i.e. there is chance to affirm people's increases in physical activity whether they are near guidelines or not, with the intention of helping clients continue with those changes. Which do you prefer?

'You walked ten minutes? so that's a hundred per cent further than last week!'

Or:

'OK so you're walking more which is good but the guidelines are 10,000 steps a day so we really need to get you doing more'

How awareness can be raised around physical activity levels in your client

Physical activity levels have undoubtedly declined. The massive increase in labour saving devices, the reduction in number of manual labour jobs and the massive increase in the number or people owning cars, means that energy expenditure is almost certainly massively reduced on a population scale. Our cars open with a click so we need not go to the effort of twisting a key, our houses are kept at a constant and alterable temperature so we need not go to the calorific expense of thermo-regulating for ourselves: vacuum cleaners replace the need for sweeping and electric mixers do the mixing- you get the idea. So the environment we live in has changed alongside physical activity levels over the last few decades and probably not un-coincidentally type II diabetes, heart disease, obesity and cancers have increased. We are not suggesting having a more luxurious lifestyle is a bad thing, or that we should go back to beating rugs and cold houses. This reduction in energy expenditure, however, does go some way to explaining the situation we face in terms of weight. Arguably, some of this reduction in the burning of Kcalories also needs replacing.

There are guidelines for how much we should do, what type of activity and the intensity needed to confer positive benefits to our health. I have worked with these guidelines for many years and still see a use for them. Although, that being said, Small Changes and indeed effective behaviour change will happen irrespective of the guidelines. The trouble is that, without being asked for, guidelines are a way of telling people what to do - and they very often don't like it.

Also there is the danger of a guideline that is so far away from the current reality (e.g. going form doing no physical activity to 60-90 minutes a day) that the client is put off (even if they were receptive to the idea of being given a guideline). So starting with where the client is, ensuring you are talking to someone who *wants* to talk about physical activity and affirming *any* kind of increase in physical activity to a person who moves around more makes a lot of sense.

Examples of tools used for raising awareness and promoting physical activity

Remember the focus (as in all sessions) should be on what the participants feel they *could* do and would *like* to do, rather than what you as a professional feel they *should* do. In essence a client can see that they do something (everyone is doing something however little) and this can be built upon.

Steps

A good example is 'steps'. Steps are fairly cheaply and easily measured with pedometers. Steps can very often be increased most easily. *It is the most readily repeatable type of activity available to most people* and obviously the client who walks only 400 steps a day then doubles their walking by doing 800 something which clearly needs affirming in your client.

Pedometers

Pedometers seem to be one of the most effective tools for encouraging physical activity in Small Changes. Walking is familiar, free and by making the small change of increasing it, big differences can result. Journeys with purpose e.g.

shopping, visiting family, sightseeing with friends, seem most popular in our experience.

Tick- list

You can also provide a 'tick list' hand out of activities where participants tick off the ways in which they are active. This can reduce their feelings of being idle and lazy as they realise that all movement counts and nearly everybody does at least some. A session should give participants awareness of what they do now and allow them to consider potential ideas for new activities they could try later.

In terms of raising awareness a physical activity pie chart is something we very often use in practical sessions. The idea is simple; a pie chart (see figure 1) is divided into four, each segment represents 6 hours of the day. Each segment is to be coloured in. Red for sleeping/lying down and being completely sedentary (say watching TV for instance) Amber for ironing, doing day to day tasks washing up and being on your feet etc. Finally Green is recorded where the client does purposeful activity: mowing the lawn, digging, climbing stairs, walking briskly or doing an exercise class. The effects of this are often that people see with clarity what they do in an average 24 hours and they also make a judgment on how active they are. In essence they become aware of their own current activity levels.

Each segment represents six hours of the day.

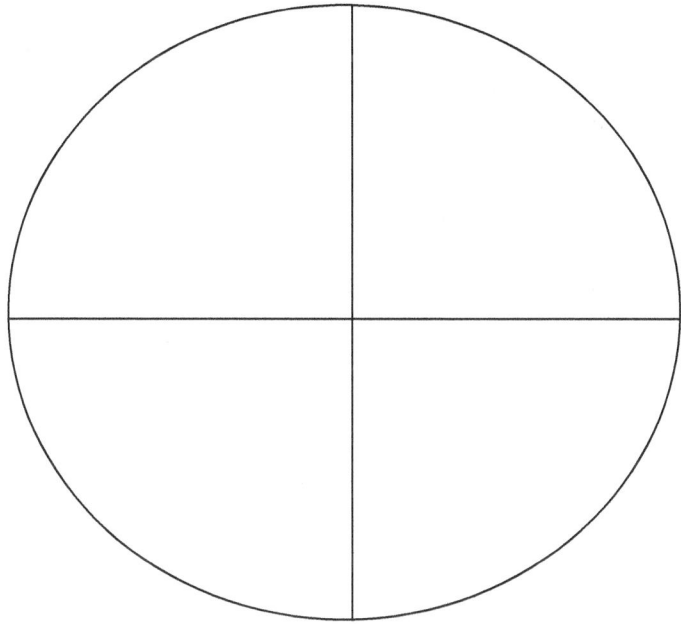

There are cleverer, perhaps more accurate research tools like the International Physical activity questionnaire to use with clients, but the pie chart is an excellent way of developing your own/a client's awareness of how much they do rather than a highly precise research tool. The idea is that as clients sit and reflect and colour in the segments of the chart they gain an awareness of how active and inactive they are. Some of the activity might be purposeful exercise, classes or walking the dog for instance and then some will be what researchers refer to as non-exercise energy thermogenesis or NEET this is the almost insensible use of energy by pottering about, walking to the photocopier maybe taking the stairs; just being active but not necessarily with dumbbells or lycra!

When awareness is raised in this way it opens the door for more exploration: *'What do you make of your own pie chart?' 'What are your thoughts about this?'* Very often followed by *'there's a lot of red on mine!'* This may even lead to plans for being more active. This choice and responsibility is of course the client's.

Physical Activity- how active are we?

Common Questions

- If I get fitter and fitter and fitter will I increase my life expectancy?
- How much is enough?
- Which diseases are implicated in people with low activity levels and what protection does uptake of PA offer? And what type?
- Should I avoid lifting weights?

There is some well-conducted research and evidence around physical activity and its benefits. Although some of this work tends to just use the description 'physical activity' as if everything were exactly the same and equal, other research looks at the specifics of doing aerobic (walking, cycling, running, swimming) type work or anaerobic (weights, resistance training etc.) and goes on to describe the benefits of both. Insulin sensitivity (a person's ability to process sugar and a proxy indicator for type II diabetes) for example appears to be better protected by a combination of both types of activity rather than one alone.

It's perhaps worth emphasising here that although the very fit may get a small advantage in terms of longevity the greatest benefits seem to occur to those moving from being sedentary (from Latin 'sedere' Literally to *sit*) to becoming moderately active. Physical activity is an independent risk ameliorator, in short it proffers a benefit in terms of lowered risk for disease even when the subjects smokes or is overweight, Paffenbarger (1986)   For instance for each accrual of 500kcals energy expenditure through physical activity there may well be a lowered risk of type II diabetes *even when the subjects remain overweight.*

This kind of information may well be asked for by clients and that is why we think a person with good level nutritional and physical activity training is needed on weight-management/lifestyle interventions. The crux, however, of the Small Changes approach is to help the individual become more physically active in a way that suits and attracts them. In short, a mode and type of physical activity which fits *within the context* of the client's life.

Small Changes Examples

Taken from our years of doing Small Changes they include:

> *People making individual trips from the patio to the washing line to hang out their clothes, dancing at home/classes, leaving work at lunchtime for a walk, waking to local shops, supervised gentle exercise classes, aqua-aerobics, exercise videos at home, walking up and down the stairs during the TV commercials, swimming, going to the gym, walking the kids to school, playing in the park, hiking, running, martial arts, cycling...and many, many more.*

Small Changes ideas for advice on activity

This would very much depend upon whether the client has asked for the information! If they are a million miles away from attending a gym, don't like going to the gym or even the idea of it… don't discuss they go to the gym…

However if the client says:

'I'm not sure what type of thing I'd like to do'

You could try:

'Would it help if I told what others have found useful or enjoyable?'

Or:

'Would it help if I told you about the sort of exercise that proves most popular with other clients?'

Within a discussion around physical activity we need to frame the concept of moderate or brisk when referring to exercise. One very popular way in which scientists collected information on the relative intensity of exercise was to use the Borg scale (Fig 1). This series of numbers relating to differing levels of difficulty for the subject is represented above. The scale matches up well to other measures of intensity such as heart rate, Dishman et al. (1987) and is obviously useful in the field for testing where laboratory equipment would be impractical or impossible. Also cardiac rehabilitation and GP referral professionals (me included) would use this tool in assisting monitoring intensity in patients.

Small Changes approach to advice

The key to making progress in increasing uptake of physical activity is behaviour change. When aiming work, advice and intervention at improving diet and or increasing uptake of physical activity how is this best approached?

It still seems fair to suggest that, often, physical activity advice relates to *telling* people what is good for them and or what they *should* do. A problem here is the human's resistance to doing what they are told to do! Either you need to know that you are speaking to an individual that specifically wants you to tell them what to do (and even in that case there are likely to be problems with compliance) or to take another approach. One such approach is to use your skills and knowledge a little differently focussing first on asking the individual what they want to achieve and then focussing on developing a targeted approach with them.

You can tell by the tone of this I am attempting to describe an approach that is not as prescriptive as say: telling someone they should eat Five A Day and do 30 minutes moderate intensity physical activity on most days. You might well feel they need telling this! But as an approach to ensure behaviour change there are difficulties.

Firstly does the person/people in question have any intention or desire to change the behaviour in question *you* may think they need to do so but this may have little bearing on them. So identifying where people are at seems essential to effective behavioural change. So what if they are not ready for the change? Well you need to decide what you are going to do next. So in this chapter we'll finish by identifying where people are at. To do this I'll introduce you to a concept that has become well established in health promotion over the last two decades.

The Transtheroretical (cycle of change) Change Model

This comes about from the work of Prochaska and Diclemente initially through work on smoking cessation which has since been adapted. The model is so neat and so good you may be tempted at first into thinking it is the answer to everything (in other words that's how I felt twenty five years ago when I first encountered it) It is not. It is a very useful way of looking at the position people are in, in relation to a given behaviour. Essentially he model posits that each of us in position of change in relation to a given behaviour (eating less cakes for example). These stage stages are: pre-contemplation, contemplation, preparation, action, maintenance and relapse. This is not to suggests that you have to pass through the stages n order instead you could jump straight from pre-contemplating a change to action for example. Another key feature is that maintenance is the stage which occurs when action has been going on for about six months.

Here is an example of a physical activity conversation from a Small Changes session:

> **SC**: 'Is physical activity something you want to tackle?'
>
> **Client**: 'I just feel that it would be better for me, you know, I'd feel better, it would be better for my health but I haven't the time to do it'
>
> **SC**: 'There'd be a benefit but fitting it in will be difficult'
>
> **Client**: 'Yeah, with the kids and work where is there time?'
>
> **SC**: 'I see a real difficulty here in balancing your other commitments with doing this for your own health - could you tell me what you are doing physical activity wise at the moment?'
>
> **Client**: 'I started walking the kids to the park after school a few times a week but I've stopped now the nights are drawing in'
>
> **SC**: 'there was some success then in being more active taking the children'
>
> **Client**: 'yes, two or three times a week, but when it's cold, it's already getting dark by the time we are out of school'
>
> **SC**: 'that's not going to work during the winter.'
>
> **Client**: 'I think I need to do something else at the weekends and that'
>
> **SC**: 'What do you have in mind?'

Client: *'I don't know maybe the park again but on Saturdays and Sundays'*

The important points to emphasise are that all the SC contributions are reflections or questions- no advice needed. The client is doing the work, making the decisions and is in charge of what they decide to do. You may not think a trip to the park of a Saturday morning is much but they are making a decision to become more physically active and the process is working...

Our coaching colleague Bob Griffiths warns about false barriers or 'obstacles' and suggests we must be careful to distinguish between a true obstacle and a justification. e.g. *'I don't have time'* which is different to the client above who immediately identifies specifically time is the issue, i.e. my life is busy, my commitments at work and my family mean there is little time left for exercise. This begins to explain the obstacle rather than justify why she doesn't exercise and allows space for further exploration. It's amazing how often this exploration leads to the client finding time.

Chapter assessment

Q1. It is vital that all people who are or have been obese should follow the exercise prescription of 60 minutes a day as per the guidelines laid down by the Department of Health T or F?

Q2. The general prescription for physical activity includes the message to work towards walking 10,000 steps a day T or F?

Q3. When clients sit and analyse what they, do on a daily basis, their awareness around physical activity rises and this may well lead to 'action planning' T or F?

Answers in Appendix 1

References

British Heart Foundation statistics page including the chapter on prevalence of behavioural risk factors for CHD:
http://www.bhf.org.uk/heart-health/statistics/prevention/physical-activity.aspx

BLAIR, S.N. AND Connelly, J.C (1996) How much Physical Activity Should We Do? The Case for Moderate Amounts and intensities of Physical Activity. *Research Quarterly for Exercise and Sport* 67(2) 193-205

DISHMAN, R.K. et al. (1987). Using perceived exertion to prescribe and monitor exercise training heart rate. Int J Sports Med. Jun;8(3):208-13

FENTHAM, P.H. et al. (1995). *Allied Dunbar National Fitness Survey* 1990 Sports Council

HARDMAN, A.E. and Stensel. D.J. (2003) Physical Activity and heath the evidence explained Routledge Abingdon

JAKICIC, J.M. et al. (2008) Effect of Exercise on 24-Month Weight Loss Maintenance in Overweight Women *Archives of Internal Medicine* 168(14) 1550-1559

LEE, I.M. HSIEH, C.C, and PAFFENBARGER, R.S JR. (1995). Exercise intensity and longevity in men. The Harvard Alumni Health Study. *Journal of the Medical American Association.* 273,15,

MORRIS, J.N. and CRAWFORD, M.D (1958) Coronary Heart Disease and Physical Activity of Work. *Br Med J.* 20(2)1485-1496

PAFFENBARGER, R.S. Jr. et al. (1986). Physical Activity, All-cause Mortality and Longevity of College Alumni *N Engl J Med* **314**, (10) 605-613.

SCHNEIDER, P. et al. (2006). Effects of a 10,000 Steps per Day Goal in Overweight Adults *The Science of Health Promotion* Vol 21, 2. P85-89

WING, R. HILL, A.O. (2001). Successful Weight loss Maintenance, *Annu.Rev.Nutr.*21;323-41

CHAPTER 7

HANDLING RELAPSE

Chapter Objectives to:

- Argue relapse is a natural element of change

- Identifying techniques for tackling relapse

Firstly we explain relapse in relation to lifestyle then we give tips and techniques for managing relapse.

Change is a constant part of human life. It is unavoidable. We interact, we learn, we experience, have ideas, we feel, react, challenge ourselves, we physically and mentally grow. So what is this fear and avoidance of 'change'? For phenomena so generic, it is incomprehensible that we not only avoid change, but do not believe we are capable of it.

Change is only recognised when 'relapse' occurs. The point at which we return to the way we were before we changed, we admit that there was a change, but we could not maintain it. The inference is therefore that change is unnatural, unacceptable and to be avoided.

There are moments in every period of change when we revert to the way we were. We refer to it colloquially as 'falling off the wagon', which indicates that we do have a language that embraces change. Normal eating is what we are used to, normal to us that is. Then we take up a diet and try to make that diet our new 'normal'. When this fails, we are back at the starting gate. It feels like a shameful incompetency that prompts all those self-doubts to clamber into our minds again. Are we lacking in backbone and tenacity? Are we weak characters with no real determination? Why does this 'always happen to me'?

Well, yes it does but it also happens to everyone else. It happens to people who are deliberately changing their way of life, perhaps from smoking, over eating or losing their temper. If they fail to maintain the change and return to smoking, over-eating and initiating a ruckus, they call it 'relapse'.

All the words that describe this stage of change – including the three terrible Ds - deterioration, disintegration and decline, or the softer ones like fall-back, setback and waning – suggest that something bad, something really, really bad, has happened. Not only that, the implication is that we are riddled with the disease of failure and it could be fatal.

The fact is, change is happening most of the time and reverting back to the way life used to live is totally natural behaviour. It is *part of* changing, not the opposite of changing.

Eating

Is it any wonder that people find change difficult and often give up? It is common for people wanting to improve their health and lose weight, to make many attempts over a period of years. We asked one group of eight participants how many years they had been attending weight control sessions.

The answer was 142. These women were expert weight losers. There was no method that they had not tried or considered trying. Cornflake, banana and grape diets, Atkins, raw food, reduced intake of calories, increased hours of daily exercise and boot camp. These and more were all familiar to the group. Many of the diets and regimes had 'worked'. Weight had been lost.

The private companies are successful in proving that anyone can lose weight if they want to. With the support of specially formulated drinks to substitute for real food, or ready meals with calories on the label and an imposed can-and-cannot system, their diets do work...

Going 'on' a diet

seems to suggest to most candidates that it is time-limited and the day will dawn when one can get 'off' a diet. There is usually the caveat of 'and return to normal eating.' The timespan of a diet is defined by the type of diet e.g. one so limited and rigid that it would be detrimental to your health to continue beyond a set number of months. Or the diet is defined by your chosen target weight. Depending on the company running the sessions, on reaching your target weight you are fit to be released from membership and expected to continue following the patterns of eating that you have been taught; or you can attend to be weighed to ascertain whether you are maintaining or defaulting from their system of choosing food (diet) that you have been taught.

Coming off a Diet - example

Two NHS nurses, working with a private weight loss company, invited us to facilitate their weight loss group after three months on a liquid only diet. The group had reached the stage of being turned loose into the supermarkets and back to eating 'real' food. The women were determined not to relapse and regain weight, but after three months of fortified drinks, they were afraid that food would tantalise and overcome their resolve. They said that they no longer knew what or how to eat.

These women were typical of the people who would describe themselves as having a weak will, lack of determination and unable to make changes. They had of course been repeatedly successful in achieving their main goal of losing weight with several private weight clubs, and just as successful in putting it back on, plus some.

Small Changes and the new normal

Losing weight and changing your lifestyle are two different goals. The first may be short term and temporary, the second is on-going and permanent. The way we live has been and is still effected by influences beyond our control. We are constantly responding to external change, each person making individual, personal decisions. To maintain the weight loss, it is necessary to continue making healthy choices of food and exercise. The 'normal eating' you started with has to be changed to a 'new' normal.

This is a normal that does not require you to argue with yourself over every food purchase or meal. It does not need constant vigilance, deprivation or panic over incidents in which you go back to the way you were. The new normal is as individual to each person as the old normal was.

The Small Changes approach works at this individual, personal level. Our lives are unique. Change decisions must therefore be personal to be effective.

Revisiting the way we were, is not a simple need to 'get back to normal' after stringent dieting. People who have been contentedly changing their tastes, making healthy choices and feeling good about the results, usually want it to continue. In fact they expect it to continue as the new 'normal'.

Triggers

However, people can be caught unawares by a trigger. Revisiting the way we were can be caused when one thing reminds you of another and precipitates an old reaction to an old association.

Take a cup of tea and you think 'biscuit'! No-one dunks a biscuit into a glass of water, but tea is ideal. It is also a long established cultural norm to brew tea in the morning and afternoon, offer it to visitors no matter what the time of day and have a 'hot, sweet' version ready to comfort and calm those in distress. All these occasions are triggers for the tea drinking habit –faithfully accompanied by biscuit and cake. Smokers may be triggered by coffee, or beer and wine. Meals in pubs and restaurants, or the end of a long day at work, are often associated with relaxing. Television, loneliness and boredom often lead to ritual smoking and snacking.

Cultural triggers are incredibly strong triggers. How can you not eat a slice of your grandchild's birthday cake? Is it possible to avoid pancakes on Shrove Tuesday? Each religion has its feast days when people eat together. Our traditions are maintained through food – Harvest Festival, Eid, Chanukah, Christmas, Ramadan. The food we eat on special occasions is in fact, part of our new 'normal'. It is very important to maintain our familial and cultural traditions. Bearing in mind that familial and cultural traditions are the triggers with the greatest impact. Fitting in with our social or workplace networks gives us a sense of stability and acceptance. Relatives and friends are profoundly important to the quality of our lives. These socially and culturally embedded triggers return us not so much to the way we were, but remind us of the way we are.

However, high days and holidays need not be detrimental to our health, because we can find a balance by making the choices. Small Changes make it possible for these healthier choices to become the norm. As changes are made and maintained, 'new' becomes 'usual'. We can live without and forget the 'should I, shouldn't I' dilemma at last.

Treats and rewards

We also use food as 'treats' and rewards. When we feel in a low mood we use it as a self-imposed trigger. A treat will make us feel better! If we are upset or worried, that means we need a treat that will comfort us. If we have had to work harder or faster, or have been challenged to achieve more than we felt we could achieve, obviously our reaction is a need to be compensated for our efforts. We reward ourselves. Obviously sugary doughnuts and a caffe latte offer immediate 'feedback' i.e. they taste good and offer gratification straight away, whereas a workout at the gym will be gratifying later, after you've laced up your trainers, headed for the gym and done the workout. The difference between immediate and delayed feedback causes us all sorts of problems! We discussed this with our personal finances (Jean and Trevor) and both of us would like to save money, this seems like a good idea, a long-term plan, a nest egg for the future... The problem is shiny new opportunities offer themselves up to us continuously, our life made so much better by a pair of shoes a new book, a treat...

The actual treat or reward, when it comes to food, is usually an indulgence that is not helping us to lose weight. They may be high in fat, salt or sugar, the taste of which can make us want more. And more! When the immediate gratification is over, guilt sets in, does this sound familiar? With our reflective thoughtful brain (not the one that makes the decision at the doughnut stand) we, very often anyway, want to lose weight when we are using that reflective thoughtful brain.

The idea of treats and rewards is essentially a good idea. Who does not need a boost now and then? An evening nibble is part of relaxing isn't it? Television football surely means beer? It is not the treating and rewarding that is the problem; it is the actual treat or reward. The old crisps, chocolates and cheese on toast could be replaced by something just as tempting and enjoyable. We could find new nibbles with little or no fat, salt or sugar. We could anticipate and recognise our personal triggers and be prepared.

There are other reasons for sabotaging efforts to improve our health. Stress that we feel from the family or work and financial demands can induce a low mood state. We begin to think there is just no point in trying, because something always knocks us back. We may react by doing the knocking back to ourselves. We self-harm by eating the crisps, drinking the beer, bingeing in any form. Having lost confidence in ourselves we strike out and make things worse, as though we feel we deserve to be punished and suffer.

The feeling that we need rewards, comfort, treats and recognition can be very deep rooted. Children who have not experienced 'good enough' parenting may become adults who live with a sense of loss or uncertainty. The theory of the 'good-enough mother', offered by Donald Winnicott (Jacobs 1995) in his psychiatric research, suggests that she is the 'ordinary devoted mother who lays down the foundations of health in the ordinary loving care of her own baby'. 'Good enough' mothering is equated with attentive, responsive care. It lays the foundation of our adult ability to be self-regulating, spontaneous and intelligent.

Revisiting the way we were can sometimes be a coping strategy. We return to habit that used to be relaxing. A habit that feels calming and safe. It helps us to cope, to feel normal and it defends us against the onslaught of the new. Or perhaps it simply meets a need that has been frozen inside us from babyhood A need that was never met, if as children, we did not receive that constant, ordinary loving care.

Small Changes sees a constant stream of people claiming to be 'chocoholics', 'breadaholics', 'crispoholics' and 'cheeseoholics'. But within a few weeks, sometimes only a few days, they do not meet the 'oholic' criteria. Participants reveal their food desire, as something akin to the addiction of an alcoholic. After their experience of private weight loss companies using good/bad food designation, people can feel guilty about eating their favourite food. Many squeeze around this dilemma by distorting the Small Change's shopping recommendation. They calculate that if we need at least 75% of our shopping trolley to contain healthy choices, then the other 25% can be anything else! Nothing is banned!

The declaration that you should eat what you like to eat, as often as you want to eat it, often comes from Small Changes participants who are caught in the strangling embrace of their personal cravings. At the same time they feel that it is a relapse which is made even worse when witnessed by fellow group participants.

There is a simple guideline. 'If you crave it – you cannot have it. If you can take it or leave it – you can take it – or leave it'.

Small Changes approach to managing triggers

The Small Changes approach is based on the Big Picture. If you are eating nutritious food, in the amounts you need to maintain your lifestyle and are being regularly physically active *most of the time*, then relapses are not the enormous problem you imagine them to be. They are not even relapses, but an integral part of change.

How can we avoid returning to the way we were? It does not always feel satisfying, or even a relief from whatever we are avoiding.

The first move is to identify your triggers. Draw up a Wanted poster and hunt them down. They lodge in very obvious places. They lack the intelligence to change into stronger more effective triggers and stick to the same- old- same- old. Think of that common phrase 'I always...'. It ends in an act that is so automatic you barely notice it until you catch yourself affirming to someone else that you 'always' have a cigarette with your morning coffee and with wine in the evening. You always have crisps in the car so that you can dip into the packet while driving. You always have biscuits in for the grandchildren and finish off whatever is left. You always hoover up left-over food and pick while cooking.

These are examples of 'normal' life for many people. It is unconscious behaviour and this is the key to changing it. Make it conscious. Make a list of everything that you eat at mealtimes and everything you eat standing up, or away from the dining table, or without a knife or fork. Tot up how many cups of tea and coffee you drink each day for seven days. Do the same for milk, juice and non-alcoholic drinks.

Get to know yourself and those 'always' habits. Rate them in order of your shock reaction when you realised how much you 'always'. These are your habits and you can work out what triggers them off. Socialising? Time of day? Another related activity - getting out of bed? Using the computer? Weekends? Saying goodbye? Holidays? Weariness after a working day?

There is more. Next is the 'I never...'list. It is not as interesting because the 'nevers' are so common. 'I never...drink water, eat fish, cook meals, forget to bring home takeaways, miss girlie nights out/in, eat white chocolate, buy anything but dark chocolate, miss a full English breakfast on holiday, eat a breakfast at home.'

Always and never are long-standing habits. They may have originated in childhood and rooted through puberty and maturity. Parents instilled some of these habits 'for your own good', others you were forced to adopt for many reasons, from the food in the canteen being too revolting; fear of trying something new, being forced to eat school dinners, disgusting smells such as bananas or whatever turned you off. Root them out and put them to the test.

Is fish really so repulsive? What harm can come from trying a Sharon fruit? How long is it since you tasted porridge anyway? This is all about you taking charge of your health, being responsible for balancing what you eat and drink to create the energy you need. Accept the challenge – change the always and never into sometimes.

If you have a generally good diet – fresh food, more home cooking than take-aways, as much variety as is available given your income and access to sources – avoid those habits, routines, old tastes and triggers that shoot you down. Identify them and when they set you off and you cannot resist, at least get their measure. The next time you will be ready chanting '*This* will be the last time.' 'This *will* be the last time.' 'This will be the *last time*'.

Given that there is no quick fix that you can make without surgery, to arrest your weight gain – it takes a long time to become over-weight and even longer to become obese – there *is* a formula. It is emerges in a list of what most people who have succeeded in losing weight and maintaining that loss, have done. This list is not everyone who ever tried to lose weight, but there are enough cases to suggest that there is a combination of 'fixes' that we could use for ourselves. These are the routines and habits that you can employ; the to do list as opposed to the don't do list.

Most people who successfully lose weight follow the same basic pattern

'*Eat less, move more.*' This persistent and enigmatic mantra for losing weight poses more questions than it answers.

Eat? Eat what? Eat when? How? How much? How often? Who with?

Move? Which way? How? How much? How often? When? Where? Who with?

If we could answer those questions, would we be able to lose weight? Would we be able to increase our fitness level and reduce our risk of contracting life threatening diseases?

Of course the answer is yes, we can lose weight by dieting, taking fortified fluids, using the system of green days/free days/sins, buying products from private weight loss companies, joining a gym, skipping, walking and training for sports.

All these methods may be sizeable departures from 'normal' life; life the way we usually live it based on our up-bringing, beliefs, culture and relationships; based on tastes, income and where we live. Consider the people that you know. Is there anyone who is exactly like you? Is there anyone who has the same way of doing things, reacts to everything the way you do, enjoys the same food, has the same abilities and strengths as you?

There is academic interest in the extent of a genetic factor in obesity. This is tempting to hang on to as a reason for giving up the effort to reach a weight that reduces risks of major life threatening conditions.

Prof Jane Wardle led a Cancer Research U.K. Health Behaviour Research Centre at University College London study on more than 5,000 pairs of identical and non-identical twins. The American Journal of Clinical Nutrition study found that differences in body mass index and waist size were 77% governed by genes. Prof Wardle also found that children who are overweight are likely to be overweight or obese as adults. Other researchers argue that it is not inevitable that the `fat gene' will inevitably produce obese children.

Fat gene or no fat gene, reducing weight and obesity or otherwise increasing physical activity, vegetable consumption i.e. 'healthful behaviours' is vital to health and longevity. People with a genetic disposition to becoming over weight may need more support to counteract the strong influences of attitudes and habits around food and activity laid down in childhood and adolescence. This is about the individual protecting their own health and being within the context of their own life, body shape and level of fitness have some strong genetic input; which does not mean I canot lk after my fitness and diet whilst being bigger than average.

More good news is, we *do* know how many people have lost weight and maintained that loss! These 'secrets', to use advertising terminology, have been discovered by asking individual people how they succeeded and keeping track of them over the years. Although the range of differences between people is wide, there are common denominators that apply to them all – the 'most people' principle. Naturally the range of achievement is also wide as it partly depends on the individual starting point and on personal goals.

The National Weight Control Registry

The National Weight Control Registry of America has a membership of which 80% of persons are women and 20% are men.

The members have lost an average of 66lbs (4st 10lb) and kept it off for five and a half years.

These are averages, within which there is a lot of diversity. Weight losses have ranged from 30lbs *(2st 2lb)* to 300lbs *(21st 6lb)*. The duration of maintaining this weight loss has ranged from 1 year to 66 years.

 The NWCR has also started to learn about how the weight loss was accomplished.

- 45% of registry participants lost the weight on their own

- 55% lost weight with the help of some type of programme
- some people have lost the weight rapidly
- others have lost weight very slowly over as many as 14 years

And here is the crux – most people succeed by *changing their food intake and physical activity.*

- 98% of registry participants modified their food intake in some way
- 94% increased their physical activity, with the most frequently reported form of activity being walking

How do most people do this?

- ✓ 78% eat breakfast every day
- ✓ 75% weigh themselves at least once a week to keep a check on progress
- ✓ 62% watch less than 10 hours of TV per week
- ✓ 90% exercise, on average, for about 1 hour per day

Most members maintain a low calorie, low fat diet and do higher levels of activity than previously. Maybe that persistent mantra `Eat less, move more'` actually does answer the questions?

Personal Small Changes

Small Changes participants make personal changes that fit into the context of their own current lifestyle. Every change is chosen by the individual according to what they feel is the most important issue for them. Our approach is designed to include every aspect of a participant's personal life, because every part of our lives interrelates and affects the whole. In short, real life is not consistently regular or organised. Unexpected events occur, accidents happen, schedules change and routines are disrupted.

By choosing the Small Changes that are feasible for them, the individual remains in control of their health decisions and will experience continuous success. A disruption of routine is just that, something to deal with, to negotiate around, to accept until it passes.

Case Study: relapse

We had been working with Lucy for a few months. The transcript below is a perfect example of somebody handling relapse effectively.

'It's like before I would always go for a large bar of Galaxy (chocolate) and Baileys' (Cream Liqueur) but I mean the whole bar and half a bottle! Now I sometimes have it when I shouldn't... What happens is I have a single piece of chocolate and 1 small glass and then I forgive myself. I've enjoyed it and tomorrow is another day when I can choose to have some or not'

The point here is that Lucy previously would: a) beat herself up for what she had done b)throw the towel in and rationalise that she had 'blown it' and may as well go on over consuming. Effective handling of relapse includes accepting that sometimes we are going to *'fall off the wagon'* but this does not mean that occasional lapses lead to giving up completely.

Assessment Questions

1. People feel a great sense of failure when they do not meet goals they have set T or F

2. A key technique for tackling relapse is accepting that there will always be occasional lapses T or F

3. Most people lose weight by semi-starvation diets always feeling a little hungry at any given time T or F

Answers in Appendix 1

References

JACOBS, M. (1995). *D.W.Winnicott key figures in counselling and psychotherapy* Sage London.

CHAPTER 8 Active Reflective Listening

Chapter Objectives

- Clarify how reflective listening is a very powerful 'tool' for behaviour change.

- Give key examples of simple and complex reflections.

Listening and hearing

Listening is a very individual process. It can be done in the company of other people in an audience at the theatre or cinema for example. Although each person may feel part of the listening crowd, listening is not a shared activity. Every individual hears, absorbs and translates on a very personal level.

Working with people seeking help on personal issues such as weight, requires more from the health counsellor than simply listening and hearing. There has to be an interaction between the health counsellor and the client that integrates both people.

The integration begins at the first point of contact, either with a letter sent to offer an appointment, a telephone call before the meeting, or a client entering the room. The effectiveness of this counsellor/client relationship rests on the initial seed of rapport planted at these first encounters.

If mutual respect can be established between the counsellor and the client, their interaction will have a foundation to support the work they expect to do together.

'Active reflective listening' is a description of the health counsellor's response to what the client says. This way of listening is intended to demonstrate that the client's words have been heard and more importantly, have been understood. That is the first level of listening. On another level, the counsellor hears more than words of information; she also hears the subliminal messages and feelings invested in them.

A common counsellor mistake

> **Client**: *'I felt so nervous this morning that I nearly didn't come to see you. '*
>
> **Counsellor**: *'There is nothing to be nervous about; we are just going to talk.'*

The counsellor speaks from her own standpoint, neatly disparaging the risk her client has taken, dismissing it as the client's mistake because there is no reason to feel nervous. She also missed the fact that this woman actually surmounted her fears and must therefore need and expect support.

The counsellor may have thought that she was being reassuring, but in fact she had made an assumption and spoken without checking that she was correct. The assumption, that the client had felt nervous about their meeting and what would be expected of her, was mistaken. The counsellor did not consider other causes of the client's nervousness

The client may have been worried about driving to a new area; the bus coming on time; her knees giving way if she had to walk too far; whether her choice of clothes would give the wrong impression, if she would remember to turn off the gas cooker... The client may indeed have been nervous for the reasons the counsellor assumed, but a general cover-all response would have been more productive.

'It can be nerve wracking, but you made it!' would have been accepting of the client's feelings and affirmation of her courage to make the journey. It would have avoided dismissing her nervous feelings as misplaced and unnecessary. It would also have avoided increasing the client's nervousness if it actually *was* the 'talk' she was worried about. This is an affirming response, relating to the client's action and would have covered all possibilities.

There is never enough information in the client's opening phrases for a counsellor to come to any conclusions. In this example, the counsellor has listened and heard the client's first words, but those words posed more questions than answers.

Is the client mentioning her nervousness as a warning that she might not stay, or she might not return for the next appointment? Is she talking about her nervous feelings because they are constant and so bad that she rarely leaves the house for fear of panicking? Is she mentioning the small matter of nervousness because she is not ready to reveal the most important issue until she trusts the counsellor? Is she trying to avoid breaking down into tears and again going through the grief that is not getting any better as the months go by? Is she chattering on because her memory is fading and she can't quite remember what she has come for? Is she simply embarrassed in front of a stranger?

Hearing listening is simply not enough to get the results the client and the counsellor are working for.

Small Changes approach to listening

Participants come to Small Changes courses with 'hand luggage', which they 'place on the table'. This luggage is the metaphoric, emotional baggage of their lives, collected through years of successes, catastrophes, losses and gains, pleasures and pains. It will be unpacked at a point where the owner feels heard *and* understood; when they are confident enough in their own ability to manage the outcome.

Simple reflective listening

Active reflective listening is a responsive method that keeps the client in charge. It involves the counsellor in paying attention to what participants say and what they do not say, how and when they speak, how often and for how long they speak. It necessitates meticulous consideration of what these things mean.

When a counsellor offers spontaneous advice and information, seeks information that they think is necessary for them to understand the issues, the client's progress is stunted. Offering opinions and conclusions harms the client's progress, are detrimental to their confidence and an assault on their sovereignty.

In the handbag that has been placed on your table, are expectations that include your interest and care for them, being treated with respect and a learning experience that will support them to take responsibility for their own health .The one most fundamental expectation is – that they will be able to describe their situation *as they see it* and the counsellor will understand and accept *their* priorities.

If a facilitator asks for specific information that will provide a starting point of the counsellor's choice, the counsellor has taken control out of the client's hands. The counsellor is then in charge.

A client has at least an inkling in her mind of which issue she wants to talk about and her introductory comment that will signal this priority to the counsellor.

The initial opening 'How have you been getting on after the wedding?' by the counsellor, wrests the client's attention away from her issue and onto the wedding. The counsellor has again made an assumption about what is the client's most important issue and taken control. The client is redirected, away from her priority issue by this chatty, incidental opening question.

The client whose courage in over-coming her nervousness was affirmed by the counsellor, with the assurance that arriving for the meeting was a good outcome for both of them, would then have been able to follow up the reasons for her nervousness.

Example of a simple reflection

Sylvia: *'I have just moved to Thistown to be nearer my daughter. Her dad died a couple of years ago – we were in Thattown, about ninety miles from here. I stayed on. Didn't really want to leave our house. We bought it when we got married and never moved. I suppose I tried to keep to the old routine so as I wouldn't miss him so much. But I have missed him every day, even with my friends coming round, keeping me going'.*

SC: *'I see - after your husband died you didn't want to leave your home – your friends kept you going and you tried to keep to your old routine – but you eventually decided to move nearer to your daughter'.*

The counsellor has briefly summarised the factual information given by her client. By repeating the main points she is demonstrating how closely she has and will listen. The 'I see' or 'I understand' suggests that she empathises with the client in her situation. She has not judged the client's reactions or decisions.

Example of a complex reflection

Client: *'That's right, my daughter, her name's Anna, said it would be easier for me to see the children. We loved going down to see them – having the car meant we could go regularly. I wish I had learnt to drive. The other thing is – I was born and bred in Thistown! It's changed a lot of course, a bit confusing with the shops all changed around. It's* *funny...for the first few weeks here I felt quite nauseous when I went into the town. Like my life had gone in a circle and I was back where I started.'*

Counsellor: *'Just let me get this right Sylvia...you have a two grandchildren here and you obviously love to see them. You used to feel very familiar with this town, being born and bred here, but it's unfamiliar in some ways now. You notice the changes made during the years you were away and going into this town centre here makes you feel sickly. It sounds as though you are happy in one way, but upset in another. Can you tell me more about that?'*

The counsellor is now reflecting on the feelings, rather than the facts, that Sylvia has described.

At the start of the session Sylvia set the scene – the events that led to her being in Thistown. She mentions the bereavement but only talks about missing her husband when she is explaining why she stayed in Thattown and the support she had.

At this point she moves into a deeper more revealing area. She is happy to be with her grandchildren, but does not understand the other feelings she experiences. They are contradictory and inexplicable to her. She may feel that they threaten her new life in Thistown and she cannot move back to Thattown.

The counsellor has summarised the feelings Sylvia shared and these were the major part of what Sylvia said. The counsellor is inviting Sylvia to look more closely at these feelings and think about how they affect her and where they may originate. Eventually, as her understanding grows, Sylvia will choose ways of dealing with the situations in which they are triggered.

It would be a mistake for the counsellor to offer her own views, to explain how normal Sylvia's feelings are (they do not feel at all normal to Sylvia) or to suggest ways of managing them. The client must always be left in control to make her own choices and decisions.

While the handbag sits on the table, there is a suitcase that has been placed underneath the table. It contains the deeper, more serious life affecting incidents in a participant's history. Old traumas in times when she felt defenceless, her self-esteem damaged, periods of erosion to her confidence and buoyancy.

The contents of this suitcase may never reach the table top. They are memories that the client may have forgotten or actively subdues. She may remember quite clearly, but not be able to talk about them. Inevitably the effects of these past experiences will influence many of a participant's present choices and decisions.

If a participant seems to be making a 'bad' decision, you can be certain that her other choices are much worse. Small Changes works on the assumption that each person is doing the best they can, given the information, resources and choices available to them at that moment in time.

A counsellor can never know everything about the client. Only the client knows everything about herself, but the counsellor can facilitate a greater self-awareness in the client and a realization of the choices available to her.

The context of peoples' lives is the exact area in which Small Changes works. It is therefore absolutely vital that the facilitator takes everything into account when supporting the participant to manage life changes. A Small Changes facilitator assists in maintaining progress and dealing with crisis by encouraging the participant to look at her lifestyle. They do not solve problems, make suggestions, or list choices for her.

A Small Changes participant is always the decision maker. It is the client and only the client, who can choose and make changes in her life. It is the client therefore, that does all the work.

Affirmation v praise

A simplistic way of differentiating between praise and affirmation is to consider whether the words refer to the feelings or opinions of the speaker.

'Good boy!' 'Well done!' 'A round of applause for you!'

These express the opinion of the speaker. The speaker thinks that the client has done well and other people would agree with her enough to express this by giving the client a round of applause. They admire and congratulate the client.. What the words do not do, is describe the action or the effort made by the client as admirable and worthy of praise. The client may then feel that she has gained the counsellor's approval and that this approval is the value of her action i.e.

the client's success depends solely on the approval of the counsellor.

Affirmation

What does affirmation refer to? clarity over what has been done or a positive quality in another person: 'You won that race in record time.' 'You said you would drink a glass of water every day and you have done' 'You have exceeded your personal best.'

Affirmations state facts about the client's actions. They described what the client did. She achieved something that can be measured e.g. won a race that had not previously been run in so short a time; challenged herself to drink water more than she was used to and succeeded; she surpassed her previous best performance.
These words are clearly not just the 'opinion' of the speaker because they describe what the subject has done. They corroborate and authenticate her actions.

Conclusion

Whole careers and livelihoods are built on the adulation of the masses. The cult of 'celebrity' demonstrates how precarious the survival of the human psyche is, when it depends on external validation.

Of course we like to be liked. We go further than that in using the admiration or admonishment of others as a measure to compare with our own internal sense of 'worthy' or 'unworthy'.

Both praise and affirmation are useful tools in weight-management. Participants need support and evidence of success to build their confidence. They are aiming to take control of their own health, to make their own decisions and to reach the personal goals they set.

To achieve this self-management, appraisal is more useful and effective than praise. Appraisal underlines what *they* have done well. It describes what *they* have succeeded in doing. It leaves no doubt that *they* took action and Small Changes were made.

Praise has a place as a common usage tool. It is familiar. Although the emphasis is on someone's opinion, we still like the feeling of being complimented. When working with people who feel they have a long way to go in changing their lives, appraisal can be internalized and used over and over to strengthen confidence and build success upon success.

Sympathy v empathy

Clients share experiences that can arouse a strong feeling response from their counsellor. The urge to comfort and console a client is instantaneous. It is part of being human to react to another person's pain.
Sympathy is often the counsellor's first reaction to the client's story, if she considers that it must have been a terrible ordeal to go through. She imagines how it would feel to be in her client's position, how hard it would be for her to recover.

She is compassionate and sensitive to the client's experience. She feels sympathy and wants to take care of her client. This response is natural, but not helpful in the counsellor/client relationship. There is a danger that the counsellor's sympathetic feelings will prevent her from helping the client to look at what happened to her. Both of them will begin to feel overwhelmed by the circumstances.

Empathy

Empathy is the feeling of 'knowing what it is like...' to have been in a similar place, or can imagine being in a similar place, to that which the client is in. The counsellor may or may not have experienced a similar trauma , but understands the effects such traumas have on the victim.

The counsellor is not re-experiencing the event, she is remembering/imagining it. She is empathic, but she stands outside the client's experience and can therefore keep a clear perspective. The counsellor can enable the client to look at her situation because she is not caught up with either her own or the client's feeling reactions. From this perspective the client and the counsellor are able to work together.

In MI four levels of reflection are referred to these are:

- Repeating
- Rephrasing
- Paraphasing
- Reflection of Feeling

Client: *'I just can't carry on like this − it is one thing after another. I get on top of one piece of work and they give me two more. I have a family, it's not possible to do all these things at the same time. I just need to get rid of some of it.'*

Repeat: *'You can't carry on like this.'*

Rephrase: *'This is too much for you, you have too much work on and you also need time for your family'*

Paraphrase: *'It's too much to have all this work put upon you as well as looking after your family - something needs to give.'*

Reflection of feeling: *'You're overwhelmed.'*

In a repeat of the client's words we are showing that we are listening to what they say and this may help them to move on with their story. In a rephrase essentially we are checking that we understand what is being said and again showing that we are listening. Paraphrasing, probably, works best with longer statements but again can help to clarify that we have understood N.B. If we have this wrong the client will correct us. Finally a reflection of feeling, offers the most complex level of reflection as here we are not merely repeating the words that have been said but rather seeking to identify how the client *feels*.

Assessment Questions
1. What are the two main types of reflective listening?
2. Which of the two refer to the client's feelings?
3. Giving unsolicited information and guidance is an effective way of helping a client T or F?
4. Praise demonstrates that the counsellor approves of the client's actions T or F?
5. Affirmation is the statement of a factually observed positive attribute in the client T or F?
6. Which is the most effective response to a client's narrative, sympathy or empathy?

Answers in Appendix 1

References

ROGERS, C.R. (1961) *On Becoming a Person A therapist's view of psychotherapy* Constable London.

ROSENGREN, D.B. (2009). *Building Motivational interviewing Skills a practitioner workbook*, Guildford: New York.

CHAPTER 9

Setting up your programme and training for weight-management

In brief

In this chapter we will attempt to sell you on the idea of supervision, give a suggestion for a one-year protocol for running a weight-management programme (do it guys - stop with the 12 week programmes already... it needs longer input to secure permanent change see refs at end) we will also discuss courses and training for weight-management workers and the ideas of developing support amongst participants during the year they will spend with you.

An example: The Small Changes Protocol

In this section we re-produce a 'protocol' i.e. a suggested way to run a programme which we used in practice. The protocol describes a one year weight management project. The idea here is to outline measures and an approach that have proven useful in gaining positive results (the one year programme has since run and is due to be published in 2014) for weight management and other measures.

Supervision

Supervision is ubiquitous in 'helping' professions and should be! supervision is not a negative top-down process where a superior points out faults... supervision is where the counsellor reflects upon her practice or his practice with the guidance and facilitation of an experienced counsellor.

Supervision allows the counsellor to develop to grow to solve problems with and enhance their practice.

As a colleague (Dr Jeff Breckon a motivational interviewing trainer and academic) said to us recently: *'practice does not make perfect- it makes consistent'*.

If you train or practice one of the major talking therapies or are a counsellor/psychotherapist you will undergo and continue to undergo supervision. At Small Changes we practice supervision with team members supervising each other and using the very same skills they use with clients to help each other develop and grow as counsellors.

The example included is suggested for running a research programme - if the research element is not what you want, keep the bits you do want and discard the rest, although it makes no sense to not include at least some measurements for the purpose of evaluation. We recognise that not all programmes will have the facilities or access to all the measures suggested below, weight, height, waist and hip circumferences, diet and physical activity diaries are at least inexpensive to produce.

The unique Small Changes unique one-year treatment plan protocol has been developed on the basis of documents provided by NICE, analysis of academic research literature and the experience of nutrition, physical activity and counselling experts involved in the programme

Methods/recruitment and approach

Overweight (BMI= 25-29.9 KG/M^2) or obese (BMI= 30-39.9 KGM^2) participants are invited on to a Small Changes course via press advertisement. Whichever category participants are in relative to their BMI the approach remains the same. The Small Changes approach is to work with clients *within the context of their own lives*. This means that despite having guidelines for eating, physical activity and lifestyle behaviours, 'context' is essential. Context means that where a client is struggling for example, with insufficient social interaction, it will be this problem that is focussed on as a vehicle for improving their life and allowing them to gain opportunities to alter physical activity patterns and dietary practices.

Recruitment and sample size

A large percentage of the population are overweight or obese. Recruitment for this pilot study will be achieved using the press advert method. In terms of study design, an outcome of clinically significant ($p=<0.05$) weight loss of 5-10% of starting bodyweight maintained at one year is suggested. Initially two groups of 20 will be recruited. Four groups of ten i.e. 2 for for each arm (experimental versus control) will mean the target of 40 'treated' people will be reached in one year.

Randomisation

A computerised randomisation package will be used to assign participants to one of two treatment groups: either the one-year protocol or the standard 3 month protocol. Participants will be randomised into blocks of ten. All participants will be measured at 0, 3, 6, and 12 months. 'Drop out' participants will form a third arm: data from this group will be analysed to examine trends of non-compliance.

Population/ exclusion criteria

The population will be adults >18years with a BMI between $25KGM^2$ and 39.9 KGM^2. Participants will be excluded from the trial if they fall outside these categories, have a diagnosed eating disorder or co-morbidities needing specialist medical treatment (eg, uncontrolled angina).

Procedure

After obtaining informed consent, participants will have height, weight, waist circumference, hip circumference blood pressure and body-composition measured. Participants will complete the General Well-Being Scale and a 3 day estimated household measures diet inventory/diary. A description of each is outlined below. The first appointment is a meeting to obtain a 'history' prior to the start of Phase 1: a 12-week 'course' that lasts for two hours each week. The first meeting is carried out at the same time and venue that the course is will take place. Participants also have their motivation to change assessed at this first meeting. This is achieved via a question asking participants to choose a phrase that most fits their situation.

Participants will spend two hours each week in sessions that use Motivational interviewing. The sessions will be facilitated by a nutritionist/ exercise physiologist trained in Motivational interviewing (the principal investigator). The facilitator will have on-going 'supervision' throughout the pilot.

Phase 1: 0-3 months

The Facilitator will help participants set realistic 'anchored' goals. The participants will be encouraged to make 'implementation intentions' which allow facilitators and participant to visualise how and when goals will be achieved. This process sets in train a plan that will help tackle obstacles that could potentially obstruct achieving that goal (Gollwitzer, 1999).

Reference to Motivational interviewing, Solutions Focussed Therapy and Neuro-Linguistic programming are common throughout the twelve-week sessions (Bandler & Grindler, 1975; Berg, 1994; Miller & Rollnick, 2002) but the approach adopted will be Motivational interviewing.

At each succeeding session the self-selected goal from the previous week is discussed, affirmation given for success or unconditional support when expectations are unmet. The phase 1 weekly topics are shown below.

Phase 1 the 12 weekly topics:

1. Introduction to Change
2. Food Content
3. Making Choices
4. Portion Sizes
5. Adapting Recipes
6. Managing Supportive Relationships
7. Mobility, Activity & Exercise
8. Talking Tough (Progress/barriers so far)
9. Alcohol
10. Handling relapses & full relapse

11. Food Mood Hunger (Triggers)
12. Affirmation (Participants' evaluation and group results)

Phase 2: 3-6 months

In phase two participants work in two-people learning sets or supportive partnerships supervised by the principal investigator. This involves participants being supported in using the techniques they have been made familiar with during phase 1.

Phase 3: 6-9 months

Meet with supportive partnerships fortnightly. In phase three the supportive partners spend three months working together with monthly meetings with the principal investigator.

Phase 4: 9-12 months

In the final phase monthly seminars take place; support using text messages (SMS) email, Skype and by telephone are also employed. The seminars allow new buddy pairs to be created where relationships have broken down or participants have decided to disengage with the programme.

Method/measurements to be used

International Physical Activity Questionnaire (IPAQ) long version

The IPAQ is a 7-day recall questionnaire which has been validated against the doubly labelled water technique and according to the National Obesity Observatory (NOO) is acceptable for estimating daily energy expenditure (NOO, 2009).

General Well Being scale (GWB)

The General Well-being Scale developed in 1972 by American Psychologist Harold Dupuy, is a well-designed, easily administered questionnaire (Veit et al. 1983). The GWB Can be sub-divided into anxiety and depression indices and offers the potential of analysing these sub-modalities in addition to a 'general' score where a high score equals positive mental state and lowers scores are commensurate with distress and negative well-being.

Resting energy expenditure (REE)

Measurements of oxygen consumption (VO_2) and carbon dioxide production will be taken to assess REE. A gas analyser and Douglas bag will be used to make the measurements using a ventilated hood system. Subjects will lie supine for 30 minutes before a ten-minute sample of air is obtained for analysis. Before each measurement a calibration will be performed using (Span Can) reference gas mixtures containing 16% O_2 and 100% n. REE will be calculated using the Weir Equation (Weir 1949).

Bio-electrical impedance analysis (BIA, spectroscopy)

Bio-electrical impedance will be used to detect change in body-composition. The tests will be carried out by using a using a body-stat 1500 (Bodystat Ltd Isle of Man) Measurements will be made on the subject's right hand side. The following guidelines will also be observed before a measurement is taken: No eating or drinking 4 to 5 hours prior to the test, no exercise 12 hours prior to the test, no alcohol or caffeine consumption 24 hours prior to the test. Right shoe right sock and all jewellery will be removed and subjects will be in the supine position. Two electrodes will be attached at the dorsal surfaces of the hand and two at the dorsal surfaces of the foot. One electrode is to be attached at the second metatarsal and the second at the posterior wrist between the styloid processes of the radius and ulna. Another electrode is attached at behind the second metatarsal and the other at the ankle between the tibial and fibular malleoli. The body stat will determine fat mass and fat-free mass. (Patients with a pacemaker will be excluded) a correlation of 0.83 has been found (Maughan 1993) between bio-electrical impedance and the gold-standard hydro-static weighing. Favourable comparison has also been made between BIA and dual-energy X-ray absorptiometry (DEXA) with results showing a high correlation between the two (r=.90, p<.05, Demura et al.., 2004) and a correspondingly high correlation in a DEXA/BIA study comparison on overweight women (r=.90, p=.001, (Erselcan, 2000).

Hydration is extremely important when using BIA for assessing body-composition as variations will alter results even when body-composition remains constant. Waist circumference, hip circumference and bodyweight measurements will therefore also be made.

Cholesterol/Triglycerides/High Density Lipoprotein, Low Density Lipoprotein via Reflotron

Cholesterol, triglycerides, high density lipoprotein, low density lipoprotein and blood sugar will be assessed using capillary blood samples. Agreement between venous and capillary samples has been identified (Bachorik et al. 1989) with correlations ranging from 0.92 to 0.96. There are, however important exceptions where values differ by a greater margin. Small Changes view the reflotron method as an important measurement for assessing cholesterol for the purposes of the study and obtaining a comparative measure, clinical diagnosis is not the intended outcome. Participants with 'abnormal' values will be encouraged to seek medical advice.

Blood pressure

Blood pressure is measured using semi-automatic sphygmomanometers. These are included in the list of validated machines by the European Society of Hypertension (O'Brien 2001). Where machines are not validated they will not be used or the protocol set by the British Hypertension Society will be employed (O'Brien et al. 1993).

3-day diet diary with training and interview

A self-administered estimated household measures diet-diary will be used. Under-reporting food intake by obese and overweight subjects has been reported previously; subjects seem more likely to under-report fat and carbohydrate rich foods than other nutrients (Heitmann & Lissner, 1995). It is therefore considerate to use dietary data as a relative rather than an absolute value. Alteration to energy intake and macronutrient/micronutrient make-up of the diet may be identified even when accurate calculation of absolute energy intake and values for macronutrients/micronutrients are not.

Waist circumference

Central fat distribution is a key indicator of risk for type II diabetes and coronary heart disease. A waist circumference of greater than 94cm for men and 80cm for women correlates with a BMI of $25kg/m^2$ or overweight. Greater than 102cm for men and 88 cm for women correlates with a BMI of greater than 30 $kg.m^2$ (Lean et al. 1995). Waist circumference is measured one inch above the umbilicus using a flexible tape measure. Investigators are trained in taking the measurements and encouraged to pay particular attention to applying the same tension on each measuring occasion.

Experience of weight-management/Small Changes

Interviews will be used to capture the experiences of participants on both this programme and others they have tried. Themes will be explored and collated form the interviews until no new themes emerge.

Measuring time-frame

Measurements will be taken at 0, 3, 6 and 12 months. 12 month. 12 month results represent an important time frame for Small Changes, continued weight loss, lack of weight gain and maintenance of healthful behaviour all represent useful data as does weight re-gain and any negative alterations to lifestyle which have been originally enhanced via the programme. For research purposes measurements beyond one year are important; anecdotal information from previous participants suggest measurements serve as motivation to maintain lifestyle change.

Statistical measurements

It is expected that ANOVA to assess the changes across the time points for measurement will be used on the anthropometric data and the $p=<0.05$ level of significance will be employed. Other tests e.g. comparison of mean values will also likely be used. Qualitative data from this mixed methods approach will be stored and analysed with the assistance of Nvivo and coded information processed for themes until no new themes emerge.

Conclusion

In this study the Small Changes one-year protocol will be examining the data for any changes occurring to the measurements outlined. Furthermore the experience of participants will be analysed and purposefully assessed relative to other programmes tried by the participants. A control group will be formed by participants who receive the standard three month protocol to observe any differences in outcomes.

Buddying/training

There are obviously loads of training courses that would be helpful to weight managers. If you've done with exercise and diet type events how about focussing on behavioural training? often the people we meet engaging in weight-management have already taken courses of training in nutrition exercise. Indeed many professional come from sport science or nutrition programmes at university and or have worked in that area for some time.

Training around behaviour change and the skills and techniques we mention in this text can be found by going on coaching and mentoring courses, motivational interviewing workshops, courses in Cognitive Behavioural Therapy. Two day and one day courses are often exciting and a great way of getting started in behaviour change. Inevitably really developing the core skills requires longer term training and supervision. You might want to refer to the BPS and CSA for further info on training. Investment of time and effort over years is needed to really develop behavioural change skills but this shouldn't stop you implementing open questions, listening skills and praising/affirming and summarising what's said to you in your weight-management sessions!

References

BANDLER, R. & Grinder, J. (1975) The Structure of Magic: a book about language and therapy. Palo Alto: Science and Behavior Book

BACHORIK PS Bradford RH, Cole T Frnaz I, Gotto Am Roberts K JR Warnick GR and Williams OD (1989) Accuracy and precision of analyses for total cholesterol as measured with the Reflotron cholesterol method *Clinical Chemsitry* 35: 1734-1739

BERG, I.K. (1994) 'Family based services: A solution-focused approach.' New York:Norton.

DEMURA, S. Sato, S., & Kitabayashi, T. (2004) Percentage of total body fat as estimated by three bioelectrical impedance analysers. *Journal of Applied Physiology*, 89(2), 465-471

DEPARTMENT of Health (2004) At least five a week - evidence on the impact of physical activity and its relationship to health - a report from the Chief Medical Officer London Department of Health

DUPUY, H,J. (1972) The Psychological section of the current health and nutrition examination survey. *Proceedings of the Public Health Conference on Records and Statistics meeting Jointly with the National conference on health Statistics. Washington D.C.: National Conference on health Statistics.*

EGGER, G. Swinburn B (1997) An 'ecological' approach to the obesity pandemic *BMJ* 315:477-480

ERSELCAN, T., Candan, F., Saruhan, S., & Ayca, T (2000) Comparison of body-composition analysis methods in clinical routine. *Annals of Nutrition and Metabolism,* 44 (5-6), 243-248.

FORESIGHT (2007) *Tackling Obesities: Future Choices — Obesity System Atlas* Department of Innovation Universities and Skills.

GOLLWITZER, P.M (1999) Implementation intentions: Strong effects of simple plans. *American Psychologist.* Vol 54(7), Jul 1999, 493-503.

HARDEN, CJ. O'Keeffe, J, Paxman JR & T Simper (2008) 'Small Changes' a behavioural change intervention for weight-management (POSTER). Tackling Child and Adult Obesity in Sheffield: Evidence, Policy and Practice.

HEITMANN, B.L. Lissner, L (1995) Dietary underreporting by obese individuals is it specific or non-specific? BMJ 311 986-989

LEAN, M.E.J, Han, TS, Morrison C.E (1995) Waist circumference as a measure for indicating need for weight-management *BMJ* 311:158-161

MAUGHAN R (1993) An evaluation of a bioelectrical impedance analyser for the estimation of body fat content. *British Journal of Sports Medicine* 1993;**27**:63-66

MILLER, W.R. and Rollnick, S. (2002) Motivational Interviewing: Preparing People to Change. NY: Guilford Press,

NATIONAL Audit Office (2001) *Tackling Obesity in England* London The Stationary Office

NATIONAL Institute for Health and Clinical Excellence (2006) Obesity: the prevention, identification, assessment and management of overweight and obesity in adults and children http://guidance.nice.org.uk/CG43

NATIONAL Institute for Health and Clinical Excellence (2007) Behaviour change at population, community and individual levels http://guidance.nice.org.uk/PH6/Guidance/pdf/English

NATIONAL Obesity Observatory (2009) Standard Evaluation Framework for Obesity Interventions. http://www.noo.org.uk

O'BRIEN, E. Waeber, B. Parati, G. Staessen, J. Myers, M.G. (2001) Blood pressure measuring devices: recommendations of the European Society of Hypertension BMJ 322:531-536

O'BRIEN, E, Petrie J, Littler WA, De Sweit M, Padfield PL, Altman D. 91993) The British Hypertension Society protocol for the evaluation of blood pressure measuring devices. J hypertens 11 (supp 2S43-S63

PAXMAN, J O'Keeffe, J Harden CJ & Simper T (2008) Micronutrient intake significantly alters when energy intake is reduced following the 12-week 'Small Changes' intervention for weight-management (POSTER). Tackling Child and Adult Obesity in Sheffield: Evidence, Policy and Practice.

PERRI et al. (1984) Effects of a Multi-component Program on Long-Term Weight Loss Journal Of Consulting and Clinical Psychology vol 52, No 3, 480-481

PERRI et al. (1989) Effect of Length of Treatment on weight Loss Journal of Consulting and Clinical Psychology, 57, 3, 450-452

PERRI et al. (1997) Effects of Four Maintenance Programs on The Long-Term Management of Obesity Journal Of Consulting and Clinical Psychology Vol 56, No 4, 529-534

SODLERLUND A et al. (2009) Physical activity, diet and behaviour modification in the treatment of overweight and obese adults: a systematic review. Perspectives in Public Health., 129,3,132-142.

SIMPER, T Harden, CJ Paxman JR & O'Keeffe J (2008) Energy intake is significantly reduced following the 12-week 'Small Changes' intervention for weight-management (POSTER). Tackling Child and Adult Obesity in Sheffield: Evidence, Policy and Practice.

SIMPER, T[1], Paxman[1], J. O'Keeffe, J[2] (2008) Small-group weight-management programme using self selected goals improves General Well Being scores. International Journal of Obesity, May S230

SIMPER, T[1]. O'Keeffe, J[1,2]. (2009) Reduced energy intake and maintained loss of weight is observed at 6 months follow up of the **'Small Changes** Programme' European Journal of Obesity May Vol2,S2 p228.

VEIT, Clarice T and Ware, John E Jr (1983) The Structure of Psychological Distress and Well-Being in General Populations *Journal of Consulting and Clinical Psychology* 51,5, 730-742

WEIR J.B (1949) New methods for calculating metabolic rate with special reference to protein metabolism J Physiol 109: 1-2: 1-9

WING, R.R, hill, J.O (2001) Successful Weight Loss Maintenance Annual Review of Nutrition 21: 323-341

CHAPTER 10 MANAGING YOUR OWN WEIGHT

In the first section you will be able to see how Small Changes courses are structured You can consider your motivation and decide whether going it alone will suit you better than being in a group. If you decide to continue by yourself, you will find various suggestions of methods and options that will encourage you throughout nine consecutive weeks. We will also point out the pitfalls that need to be avoided in order for your progress to be smooth, enjoyable and successful.

You will also find hand-outs with information that we have prepared, which answers the questions asked in most of our groups. They are designed to anticipate your own questions as a solo participant and are listed at the end of this chapter.

There are only three pieces of equipment that you need: a pedometer, a notebook and a pack of gold star stickers.

Overview

All the Small Changes that you choose and achieve are cumulative. They are repeated every week until a maximum point is reached. This snowballing method ensures that you will be able to fit changes in as your natural, habitual choices, without colossal willpower or exhausting discipline. Following the course for a block of nine weeks, rather than taking a break of a week here and there, is important. Creating a routine develops your personal choices of change and progress to your own goal. It avoids the effort of constant 'remembering' leaving you with the realisation that this course is well within your capabilities; which of course it is.

The absence of inner debate - 'will I – won't I', 'Can I, can't I', 'Good choice, bad choice', is the foundation for your new 'normal'. The 'I always, I never' monuments of your old normal are replaced. Your taste will change and eating will not be on your mind every waking hour. You will enjoy choosing food and eating it without fear of ruining your diet., because there *is* no diet!

Small Changes participants imagine a normal life; a life free from the constant struggle with habits, defence mechanisms, comfort, boredom, addiction and self-esteem. They want the ease of being competently in charge of their health, to naturally gravitate to the nutritious foods and to lower their potential of developing debilitating or terminal illnesses.

All this is all achievable. It is your life - your choice.

Is it advisable to go it alone?

Why not? If you cannot attend a Small Changes group, or feel uncomfortable with people you do not know, or even those you *do* know, but you still want to use the approach for yourself, then this may be the ideal answer for you.

What difficulties would you face that would not occur in a group situation?

Support

If you intend to use the Small Change approach by yourself, then you will not have the same amount of support as you would within a group. Participants do find that being with others, who are facing the same issues and have experienced the effects of being overweight or obese, motivates them to keep overcoming the barriers to change. They do not feel so isolated when they can share their difficulties and problems. Small Changes groups are always enlivening. Participants feel that they can rely on the facilitators and the members of the group to give them the support they need, when they need it.

We would suggest that you set up your own support before starting. A friend, a relative, or another person who has benefited from losing weight, may be delighted to help you. You may know relatives or people outside the family who could encourage you to keep going. However, if you feel you cannot ask even the closest or most-likely-to-say-yes person, or you simply want to do this privately and you feel that you have determination, then there is nothing to prevent you being just as successful as any participant on a Small Changes course.

Celebrating success

Being in a group is useful for celebrating successful changes. Someone who does not know the approach might not think that going swimming is anything to shout about, but if you have not been to the baths for years, it is a tremendous achievement. If you usually only drink tea and coffee, but replace one coffee a day with water, you have successfully increased your water intake by 100%! That is a small change with enormous benefits.

We will give you ways of celebrating your successes privately and these will form an important record to look back on. At the end of a course, many Small Changes participants feel that they have not make much effort in relation to the success they have had, because it felt so easy to make the changes. This is exactly what we are trying to achieve, but, you *will* need to acknowledge that it was you who made all the decisions and followed through with all the changes. The records you keep will testify that you can confidently continue to use the techniques you have learnt to keep the weight off.

Shared experiences - new ideas

How can we cut down on Mars bars? Is it even possible not to eat a Mars bar that calls to you from the biscuits and sweets cupboard? A group participant informed us of an ingenious solution to this tough chocolate barrier. It is, if you cut the bar into ten slices and freeze them separately. Our participant assured the group that by taking each slice and let it defrost in your mouth, and savour the taste, you could prolong the pleasure of the bar over five or more days. For that person it was easier in this instance to cut down rather than cut out. We have also experienced frozen bananas as a substitute for ice lollies. Please remove the skin first otherwise you have a weapon rather than an ice lolly!

Skipping on the rear patio at 6am may not appeal to everyone, but one shy participant felt that the only way she could exercise without feeling embarrassed and exposed to adverse comments, was to use a skipping rope.

Following the course by yourself will mean developing your own ideas about what will work for you, just as people in the groups do. The difference is that you will not be exchanging ideas with others. However, we will share with you many of the ideas that have been brought to our attention in Small Changes groups and which were adopted by other members.

Facilitation

Small Changes three month courses are run by two facilitators. Participants, who have varying levels of experience and knowledge of health factors, can ask for any nutritional or behaviour change information they need. This might be of general interest, or may relate entirely to the individual's circumstances. If you are not in a group you will not be able to ask the questions that come up for you personally, at the moment they come up.

We will provide you with a list of frequent – and infrequent – questions asked by past group participants, plus the website address where you can email us.

Demonstrations and practice

Some parts of our three month group courses involve practicing new skills together. An example of this is a food label reading session and assessing where adjustments of ingredient intake e.g. sugar and salt, can benefit participants' health. The variety of ways that different food manufacturers print ingredients and the levels of, for example, salt content, can be very confusing. In the groups we have as much time as it takes to get to the point where everyone feels confident enough to read and understand food labels when they next go shopping. Participants (i.e. yourself in this case) really benefit from sessions such as this which are often punctuated with gasps of astonishment and cries of dismay if a favourite food is high in sugar, moans of annoyance as some struggle to get it right and a great deal of laughter as people help each other.

We support participants by giving them examples of popular food labels and clearly explaining how to read the food labels in their own cupboard. If they take the time needed to use their new knowledge at the supermarket, which generally takes twice as much time as their routine shopping takes; this necessary foundation enables them to automatically make subsequent healthy choices thereafter.

Forming relationships

Participants on Small Changes courses often form new friendships. These may continue as telephone based relationships, but if participants live near to each other and have access to the same facilities such as gyms, swimming baths, cycle paths, walks – including shopping mall walks of course, then they meet and increase their activity levels together. You may find that incentive is more difficult to conjure up and maintain if you do not have relatives and friends to join you.

Having extra contact with another group participant can result in timely boosts of confidence and determination when 'real life' interferes with your new routine. They can easily coax each other back to a routine if they are already part of it.

We will suggest techniques that will help you to assess any interruptions of your progress and ways of dealing them. If you do have support from someone you will be able to explain *exactly* how you need to be supported. People may be are well meaning but not always accurate in their support.

Introduction to Small Changes approach

The Small Changes approach can be described very simply and briefly. There are four components; raising your self-awareness, working within the context of your life, choosing personal changes and anchoring your chosen You will be able to.

Firstly, raising awareness. This is really a study of yourself. The more you know about yourself and your past, how you react to different situations and what is important to you, the more effective your chosen changes will be.

Think of those childhood mealtimes. Did you eat at the table with brothers and sisters? Did you have to eat quickly before a sibling forked food off your plate and into their mouth? Was your father a stickler for 'manners' and jumped on any child who dared speak with their mouth full, or tried to hide their most hated vegetables under the mashed potatoes? Do you remember delicious favourite meals and how you got into trouble for laughing at the naughty antics of your younger brother?

A Small Changes participant remembered teatimes with her Dad. They both read books while eating at the table. Mum worked late and when she came in was full of gossip and energy.

There were two or more ways to assess the influence of these childhood teatimes. Either the participant does not pay much attention to the delights of eating, or she is only able to relax and eat at the table if those present are few and quiet. Or perhaps all mealtimes are anticipated with pleasure and she overeats in order to prolong them. There are multiple conclusions to be drawn from any childhood experience, none of which serve as a reason to stay as you are.

However factors like these do usually influence the level of ease or discomfort adults feel around meals, buying food, or eating in public. That influence will effect your capacity for, or willingness to choose the changes that you want to make.

Your social network, place of work, culture, every experience you have had so far, has moulded your life. All the 'have to 'and 'never could 'beliefs originate in earlier experiences. They form what you feel is 'normal' for you. Your habits, desires, tastes, make up your personal, current 'normal life'.

We were not born loving chocolate and being disgusted by Brussels sprouts. It was not our 'nature' from birth to be daring or timid, but more likely experiences and examples set for us are powerful enough to develop or degrade genetic factors. If you want to make healthy changes in your lifestyle, you will need to know your strengths and what may hold you back.

Firstly, Small Changes is not about making temporary changes to increase well-being and lose weight and then you can 'get back to normal'. It is about increasing well-being, loss of weight and creating a new normal – *your* personal new normal.

The changes you make are cumulative. They continue each week e.g. increased steps recorded on your pedometer until you have reached the amount of walking that fits your lifestyle. Other changes such as eating more fruit and vegetables and drinking more water are maintained every week until they become your normal routine.

Secondly, we are working within the context of your life. This means that any changes that you want to make, must be small enough to slot into the way you live; taking into account your current responsibilities, employment, caring duties, time out and family involvement. If the change interferes with your routine to the extent that major commitments are disrupted, you will be less likely to keep it up.

Thirdly, choosing a change - if the change is too challenging, the effort and discipline needed to accomplish it will become over-powering. You will feel disappointed and angry with your apparent 'lack of willpower' and 'failure'. The following technique will help you choose and tailor some of your change decisions and is an example of the type of assistance you can expect in the Solo course.

What is your favourite food? Think of the one that you eat most, or the food that would be the very last one you could imagine completely giving up. If a renowned medical consultant told you that this food is seriously damaging your health and this frightens you enough to want to give it up – would you cut it out, or cut it down? Understanding which you are is an important awareness that will effect your progress.

You may say that your decision is influenced by that fact that the food you chose was your favourite and other foods are much easier to give up. This is true. Each decision about making a change is dependent on the food and you will be making cutting out or cutting down decisions accordingly.

The change should always be less that you imagine you can do e.g. you eat chocolate every night while watching television; it is your relaxing time; it makes you feel rewarded for all the effort you had put in during the day. Deciding to cut it out completely may result in a nightmare of temptation and misery.

If you cut the small change down a little; restricting it to two evenings per week, this is a 'cut out' decision, but is regulated so that the chocolate is still on your menu. Or you could reduce the amount of chocolate you usually eat at one sitting. This is a straight forward 'cut down' choice. It will take some ingenious planning to avoid taking just one more piece!

If you feel relaxed with either of these decisions, you will increase your decision making confidence in achieving agreed small change. Remember not to outstretch yourself. Change will become easier and easier to achieve as you go through the course.

Some time ago, a health promotion campaign placed notices at the foot of railway station escalators. The notice informed commuters that if they took the stairs instead of the escalator they would be using X number of calories. CCTV cameras showed that over a period of time 70% of commuters used the stairs rather than the escalators, as opposed to the previous 5%. This is a perfect example of fitting exercise into the context of your life.

Sadly, there were subsequent lessons to learn. When the notices were removed, a proportion of the 70% on the stairs, reverted to using the escalators. Either the notices were not there long enough for the habit to be ingrained, therefore demonstrating that repetition is essential; or if there is no 'reminder' for commuters, the change may be forgotten and never becomes the new norm. Fridge magnets spring to mind, but be inventive and think of something that would constantly gain your attention and remind you to keep your Small Changes going.

Another of our participants had just started to drink water and was not only feeling the benefits, but began to enjoy it. He wanted to drink more water but just could not remember to do it. He admitted that he only drank water before breakfast and when eating during his lunch break. After his evening meal he spent hours upstairs on the computer. Even more time was devoted to the computer at weekends.

A fellow member of the group suggested that he took a jug of water upstairs, put it on the computer table where he could see it and poured it into a glass as soon as the glass was emptied. This anchoring had all the advantages of a prompt and very easy access within the context of his computer activity.

It produced great results too. The participant began to notice when he had not had a drink of water for a period during the day. He became aware of his thirst and realised that he had become dehydrated. To avoid dehydration he needed to be drinking water more regularly. Making sure that it was at hand meant not waiting until he became thirsty. His new norm had been established.

Other tastes, such as salt, will change as you make Small Changes. Reducing a high intake of salt and sugar very soon creates a sensitivity to the taste, which leads to further reduction of intake. A little salt or sugar goes a long way when you are using less than you were used to.

Which small change to choose depends on what is most important or urgent to you. The question is about priorities. One health factor may be causing you more concern than another. You may worry about being inactive, or constant snacking, using too much salt or feeling addicted to sweet foods. You are faced with two questions. What do you feel you need to do first? How easy or difficult will it be to make a change in that area?

Fourthly, anchoring your 'you will be able to'. When a small change has been decided upon, the next important consideration is to detail the 'you will be able to'. How can you ensure that you will repeat the you will be able to? This is another facet of working within the context of your life. By looking at the details of where the 'you will be able to' will take place, what time that will be, how often, who else will be there, how long will you do it, will visitors, the weather, or other responsibilities get in the way? Make a note of your answers to these questions. Be as clear as you possibly can. Repeat the what, where, when, how, who with and how often answers until there is no doubt in your mind about completing the small change.

Make it absolutely concrete. It is important that there are no other decisions to make, nothing to discuss with yourself or leave to your mood at the time. There is no 'will I, won't I' or 'leave it till another day' to waste your time with anxiety.

One of the advantages you will have from going it alone, which the groups do not have, is that when you have completed the course, you can continue with the changes you have made with the support you have in place. There will not be the feeling of something ending and being alone again, which many participants feel very keenly after what they see as a changing experience. In our experience, continuing personal support after a course ensures that a participant will not feel that being 'on their own' sensation.

The weekly sessions are carefully co-ordinated to allow sufficient time for 'living' the theories and embedding the changes. As a solo participant you should avoid the temptation to collapse two or more weeks together, simply because you could. You could name your version Explosion of Changes!

Small means small in size and small in sequence. Each week you will have a new experience, essential for framing your 'new normal'. These are in the order that leads to more success than any other we have tried. Getting used to your chosen change takes at least one week and adding one more change to your routine every week takes concentration and inner conversations of encouragement with yourself.

Changes that are maintained cannot be made out of sequence or in combination. Try not to be tempted to adapt the course because it feels easy and slow and you want quick, big results. Avoid reading ahead and planting new thoughts in your mind before the last one is safely rooted.

We offer the same advice to you as to group participants. Maintenance of change is vital until it becomes your 'new normal'. At the point where you are not thinking about how much and what you eat, whether you are active enough, if your weight is going up or down, needing more support; you are then living your new, healthier *normal* life.

Sustaining this may need a boost in the months following the course. If you begin to feel less energetic and confident and more worried, go back and use the techniques that helped you to change. Keep a food diary again and check what, when and how much you are eating with the food diary. Use your pedometer for reassurance that you that you are still active enough.

Think back on the tips that worked for you. Remember how you successfully tackled difficult issues – do it again. Ask your support person to remind you how amazing you have been at keeping going, how fantastic the results. Try not to waste time regretting lapses or interruptions. Real life happens and it can get in the way. There will be periods when other things are hugely more important that a hiccough in your attention to health. Have a good moan about the problem and then say SUMO – shut up and move on!

Pre-course preparation

Choose the week you want to start the programme, preferably a week hence, at a period which suits your timetable. This gives your conscious and unconscious mind time to start working and for you to become familiar with the idea of concentrating on yourself. You may begin noticing health indicators. It is similar to being pregnant, or buying a Mini. Suddenly every third woman you see is pregnant and every second car is a mini. Or you may begin to notice more people who look very fit, or who are obese. The main point is that anticipating the start of your time to improve and enjoy your health and fitness, results in an effortless mental preparation. Just be yourself and it will happen naturally.

Week 1 Start up & support

This week is a prompt and practical preparation, designed to familiarise you with the Small Changes method of working. In subsequent weeks you will get to know the approach we use and begin to practice it, but for this first week – simply anticipate starting on a course that can change your life. Let this idea run around in your head and you will find yourself very well prepared for week two and beyond.

You should be able to:

- source and purchase all the materials you need to take you through the whole course
- be aware of the way these will be used
- use the pedometer to record your usual number of steps
- fill in your food diary for seven consecutive days
- understand the importance and effect of using the materials
- gain an overall impression of the input required of you
- realise that it is essential to keep to the approach and timing specified
- keep strictly to your normal daily routine and social life
- experience the start of self-awareness and a subconscious build-up of anticipation

Week 1 Action

Resisting the temptation to start at Week 2, or to do Weeks 1 and 2 in tandem, reserve this week to buy a small notebook that will be easy to carry around. Buy one with a design and colour that appeals to you, because it will become very precious. In it you will record your progress.

Because Small Changes slip easily into your life and because you will not be criticised or driven to make more effort, you may feel as most of our group participants do – that you have not made any great effort at all. Your notebook will prove otherwise, so keep a detailed record of your Small Changes, successes and reYou will be able tos. It will be important to acknowledge your progress and feel justifiably proud of yourself. Knowing that you are responsible for your own health and can manage it successfully, will ensure that you will weather the interference of 'real life'.

Purchase a card or two of coloured, shining star stickers. These stickers are also an evaluation tool that you will find useful.

Buy yourself a pedometer too. The very basic ones that simply record your steps are sufficient and least expensive. Keep strictly to your usual routine and record the number of steps you do each day. You can work out an average by adding them up and dividing by the number of days you recorded - anything from 2 – 7 days. This will give you a starting baseline figure from which to compare following weeks' steps and raise your awareness of how much you are on your feet and moving.

You might like to get weighed before you start the course, preferably on accurate, reliable scales that you can use again at the end of the course. Make a decision not to monitor your progress by weighing every day or week. Weight fluctuates and you will feel disappointed and disheartened if you have gained 'weight' and you think it is fat when it might be a development of muscle. There will be changes to your body that are significant in assessing a person's health. Weight is not the only important factor. Wait till the end of the course to weigh yourself again.

Participants on Small Changes courses often develop a waist, or reduce the size of the one they have. You can measure yours – it is on level with your belly button – and enter the measurement in your notebook.

Week 2   Self-evaluation

This week begins the process of evaluating your progress and will continue throughout the course. There are several evaluations to complete, each one will reveal different aspects of your lifestyle. They will provide the starting line that will enable you to see how much you have changed your lifestyle in order to gain the benefits you will experience by the end of the course. The writing that you will do every week, starts this week.

You will be able to

- begin to notice and make notes on your feelings and responses to increasing your self-awareness
- experience the discipline needed when going solo, to follow instructions, keep to the one-week-at-a-time and not read ahead
- question your efforts to be honest, even when your answers *are* honest
- begin to establish your own daily timetable for the course
- include the two stipulated Small Changes for the following 7 days

Week 2 Action

- Write a couple of lines in your notebook diary that describe how you feel at the start of Small Changes – excitement, dread, panic, relief?
- List your very favourite foods. Choose one of them and underline it.
- Put yourself on the two Rating Scales by circling one number on each scale that represents how motivated and how confident you feel at the start of this course.

- Look at the Mountain handout. It represents your health journey. The top of the mountain being at the peak of good health, the foot of the mountain being the point at which you feel you are starting. In between the two are various points that you may feel you have reached already, but are not quite as high as you would like to be. Mark the point where you feel yourself to be this week. Write in your notebook your reason for choosing that point.

- In your notebook, write the question 'Do you eat three meals a day?' Answer Yes or No if that is regularly, or mostly yes/no if meals are irregulart. A meal in this instance is eating either sitting down, using a knife and fork, or spoon if it's soup, or any other hand food that you class as a meal ie not a filler/snack - crisps, nuts, biscuits, sweets, dried fruit, cake, biscuits and chocolate.

- Write in your notebook the number of teas, coffee, milk, juices, flavoured water, Lucazade, coke, fizzy pop, Bovril, chocolate, cocoa, Ovaltine, Horlicks that you drink per day. Start drinking water if you do not drink it already or more water if you do. If you drink water at all this week - well done!. Read the handout on drinks.

- Record on your food diary what you ate and drank yesterday. Just the food and drink, not the amount. Fill this in every day because it will help you notice the range of food you eat, how often and at what times. This comprehensive view is information you can use to make healthier choice changes. It is also another way of recording the progression of your successes.

- If, after an examination, an eminent consultant told you that the favourite food which you underlined in your notebook, was a risk to your health and would result in severe damage if you continued to eat it...... in an effort to reduce the risk would you cut it out, or cut it down? Record this answer in your notebook.

Making a Small Change At Week 2

- Keep your food diary

- Replace a tea or coffee with a glass of water

- Continue to use your pedometer and record your steps

NB. Collect labels of food you eat e.g. cereals, biscuits, ready meals, sauces/relishes, anything that shows ingredients and levels of sugar, fat and salt, to use next week.

WEEK 3

Food Labelling

Star check

If you kept your food diary, used your pedometer, recorded your steps, and drank more water than usual, award yourself three stars. Stars are available from stationary shops and anywhere that sells art and craft stuff, stick them in the front of your notebook, or inside on a page reserved for stars. Make sure that the first three or four pages of your book reserved for stars! This slightly infantile sounding activity has profound effects in our experience so just humour us nd give it a try.

This week takes a close look at the fat, salt, sugar and other contents of processed food. It will enable you to assess how much fat, salt and sugar you are swallowing each day and compare it to the daily allowances for women and men.

You will be able to

- learn and practice how to read food labels
- note comparisons between different brands
- assess your own intake compared to the recommended daily amount
- decide on where you could most easily lower your intake of fat, sugar, salt

Week 3 action

Working with food labels can be quite an eye opener, if not a direct shock, but it does give you the skills to make informed choices about how much fat, salt and sugar you are consuming. It is more useful, if at the beginning you look at your own food labels – the things that you eat on a regular basis. You will then have an idea of which ingredient you would like to reduce. We will provide you with information on the amounts that are high, medium or low.

By looking at other brand labels you may want to simply change brands to lower your intake. Remember to look at fat, salt *and* sugar, because in decreasing sugar, for example, the food producer may have increased the fat or salt content to make it more 'tasty'. If this discovery makes you feel that you are faced with an impossible choice, you need to decide which is the most important reduction for you. Perhaps you have a higher intake of sugar compared with fat – so your choice might be to reduce sugar.

Take the label information with you when you are next shopping for food. Our participants remark on how much longer this takes, but invariably they are able to make choices and feel more confident about what they eat. Subsequent shopping returns to the time you usually take.

The food credit card

- Notice that sugar is listed under 'Carbohydrates of which are sugars'.
- Note that on the label card the figure in the green band is a low amount of salt, fat or sugar that is recommended per day in a healthy food plan.
- In the amber band is the amount is medium and is preferable to the potentially dangerous amount in the red circle. The green band indicates the amount of fat, salt and sugar that is the lowest.
- If your food shopping basket contains mostly food in the green and amber bands, you are choosing more healthy brands. If you have many items in the red band, you could think about changing to a different brand of items with a lower content of salt, fat or sugar. You are aiming to *reduce* your intake gradually, *not* leap into the green band and have to struggle with a change in taste that is too dramatic.
- Where sodium is listed, multiply that figure by 1.5 and add it to the amount of lt.
- Using the handout, take the amounts from a label of your choice and enter them on the content comparison form. Enter several labels in this way,

especially different brands of the same food e.g. baked beans, biscuits, tinned vegetables, stock cubes and mayonnaise.

- It is possible to find brand with for instance, lower fat content, but beware that they do not contain more sugar.
- Watch out for the way manufacturers present the figures to you. Some give the amount in the whole tin, jar or carton, while others give list the amount in 100gms. The pack or wrapping design induces you to think the food is 'healthy' e.g. countryside scenes, happy people, promises of energy. ClYou will be able to of 'reduced' sugar are not backed up by the original amount – a reduction from 20gms to 15gms is not as healthy as a reduction from 10gms to 5gms.
- Cooking from scratch is another answer to avoid going over recommended levels. You will know and have control over the ingredients in the meal that you prepare.

Making a small change at week 3

Take your label information to the supermarket or local shops and use it to find out which other food choices you are using appear in the green, amber or red range.

Make one small change in your choice of processed food, remembering last week's answer on whether you prefer to cut down, or cut out, when aiming to reduce consumption.

Week 4

Fat, Salt, Sugar

Star Check

If you used your labelling information when shopping, made a small change in your choice of processed food and have increased your average steps for the week, award yourself 3 stars. You are on your way! Well done!

This week we will use your three weeks of entries in the food diary, to give you a clearer sense of direction. Now is the time to study the information in those food diaries and make change decisions in the most important areas. Importance is related to any eating, whether it's the frequency, content, snacks, non-nutritional or weight inducing food.

You will be able to

- o understand the relationship between fat, salt, sugar and life threatening diseases
- o become more constantly aware of nutritional values
- o measure the amount of salt you add to your cooking or meal
- o gain a comprehensive overview of the variety and nutritional value of your menu
- o be able to make an informed decision to make changes that will lower your risk of seriously debilitating physical conditions
- o experience the effort of carrying extra weight
- o use your food diary to increase the effectiveness of your chosen Small Changes
- o choose your own small change and anchor it

Week 4 Action

Make a list in your notebook of all the different foods you eat, grouping together meat/fish/seafood; fruits/vegetables; nuts; rice/pasta; potatoes roast/chipped/boiled; bread/biscuits/cakes/tarts/desserts; butter/margarine/spreads/dressings/oils/sauces; and put takeaways in a separate category.

a) Highlight or write in
   o red - meat and fish
   o green - fruit/veg
   o blue - rice/pasta
   o yellow - bread/pastry/cakes/biscuits and takeaways
   o
b) Enter the following answers in your notebook.

1. How many different foods do you have in each colour?
2. Are you eating a range of foods within these categories, or just one or two?
3. In vegetable and fruit category are you eating more of one colour than the others?
4. Which fruits and vegetables are you eating and which are you avoiding?
5. Which foods on your list contain the most fat, salt and sugar per serving?

c) Compare your figures with those on the hand-out 'Fat, salt, sugar levels. Do you deep fry, spray fry, grill, boil, poach, steam? Read the handout 'Cooking With Fat'

NB. You are more likely to gain the amount of nutrition you need if you eat a variety of fresh food.

Does the texture of fresh food effect your choice? Make a note.

It is recommended that we eat three meals a day, one of which has to be breakfast which kick-starts your metabolism. Regularly spaced meals will provide the energy you need during the day.

The nation is encouraged to eat at least five portions of mixed fruit and vegetables per day. Fruit juice drinks can only be counted as one portion per day.

A participant in a recent group complained that we had provided red grapes and she only like green ones. In fact she never ate red grapes because they tasted funny. Her friend insisted that there was no difference between the two colours and she should at least try a red grape.

Later in the morning the complainant admitted that she had been eating the grapes throughout the session and realised why she thought she didn't like them. 'I don't think I ever tasted one before today! I must have decided against them years ago and forgotten why.'

If there is any food that you have been averse to for as long as you can remember, try it again. Our tastes do change. Or try something new that could help you increase the variety of food you eat.

Shake a salt cellar the same number times that you do over your meal, or into your cooking during one day. Use a plain dark plate or bowl so that you can see and weigh the actual amount. Increase this by 7 to get the total amount for a typical week. Are you over the recommended limit?

Place enough tins of food into a bag or rucksack to weigh one kilo. Carry this on your back for thirty minutes. One kilo of weight requires that amount of energy and increases the demand on your heart. Add another kilo and think about how reduced the stress on your body will feel when you reduce your weight.

Making a small change at week 4

Think about your small change this week in relation to what you do, or do not eat and how you cook it. How can you improve on the present food diary pattern? Make a note in your book of your choice, with the when, where, how, who with and how often details.

Week 5
Portion Sizes
Star Check

If you have increased your yellow or green mobility area, award yourself a star! If you have increased your steps, add another one. If you have made more than one change, take a bonus star!

You will be able to

- be able to describe the origins of your present portion sizes
- estimate whether they are too large or too small
- understand the relationship between food quantity and activity
- consider the size of plates and bowls you use
- know how to produce a balanced plate of food

Action

The difficulty with the amount of food we put on a plate, is that we all think that we eat well and the right amount. No-one has ever joined a Small Changes course and declared that they ate unhealthily. We tend to eat the way we ate when our parents were cooking and serving the food. We also tend to eat much the same food and our favourite meal is often one that Mum or Dad made.

The truth is that there is a huge disparity among households. If we observe the meals that other people eat at home or in restaurants, we often make a judgement on whether they have too much, or less than we have. This is a completely subjective observation, apart from the opinions of nutritionists and dieticians of course. Compared to us, we say, their portions are huge or skimpy. We are unshaken in our belief that the amount we eat is the correct one.

We believe in a collection of myths too. Vegetables are good for us, the more the better.

See the hand-outs on Myths and the Three Bears and Perfect Portions, Food Fuel. We have provided other hand-outs on how to measure portion sizes

Take a few minutes to explore your childhood and make notes. Who cooked and served the food in your house? Was there a competition to get second helpings? Did siblings eat fast or slowly? Which meals did you love, or hate? Were you compelled to eat everything on your plate, or reminded about the starving children in Africa? Was mealtime fun or an ordeal? Were the people in your house worried about their weight? Did everyone have the same meal? Did Dad and the boys receive larger portions? How would you describe what went on during your childhood and adolescent periods?

From the notes in your notebook, pick out what you feel were the formative factors that led to your own eating habits. Which habits and choices can you trace back to your original family?

1. What has influenced your eating patterns as an adult? Social factors such as: casually eating at any time of the day, availability of fast food, the eating habits of friends, takeaways or eating out? Did your culture or religion exert any influence on your choice of food? What emotions effect your desire to eat? Have you always been able to afford to buy and food of your choice? Did having children change your appetite or create new food fads? Do you now eat the children's leftovers, or anyone else's? Did taught attitudes such as 'Waste not, want not', the impoliteness of taking the last slice of bread or cake.

2. Note in your notebook your answer to these questions. Do you think you eat too much, or too little, or just enough? Do you eat three meals a day? Do you eat at regular times? Do you eat breakfast?

Which meals do you skip? Do you always eat after 8pm? Do you eat between meals? Are you ever hungry? Do you eat whether you feel hungry or not? Does being away from home effect your eating?

3. Look back at the number of drinks you have in one day. Do these lessen your hunger? Do you use drinks to curb your eating?

4. After reading the hand-out on recommended portion sizes, do you think you need to cut yours down? One trick that Small Changes participants find successful is to use a smaller plate. This has two advantages. Firstly you cannot get as much food onto it – piling high is not an option! Secondly a fully covered small plate deceives the eye, making us assume that we have as large a portion as we are used to. Or do you need to increase your portions?

5. Eating more slowly, or pausing now and then, will help you to take more notice to the look and taste of the food. It also allows you to be aware of feeling full or not. You can then make a decision. If you want to continue eating, do so. If you feel that you have had sufficient, place your knife and fork on the plate.

6. Similarly if you chew more you can savour the taste for longer. Chewing also aids digestion and strengthens your teeth.

Making a small change at week 5

Choose a small change that involves increasing the regularity of your meals to provide energy when you need it e.g. breakfast, and two other meals; or if you think you need to reduce your portion size, start with reducing one item or reducing additions to the meal that are not on your plate e.g. bread. Devise a way to avoid second helpings.

Week 6 mobility

Star Check

If you succeeded in making a small change to your food diary, award yourself a star! If you have increased your steps, add another one.

You will be able to

- o create a clear picture of how you spend your time

- o assess where in your routine you can introduce more activity

- o choose an initial small change as a starting point or an increase of present exercise

- o understand the benefits of mobility

Week 6 action

Week five is the time to consider how active you are. Look at the Mobility Pie handout that is divided into four sections, each representing 6 hours. This marks a 24 hour period, covering one night and one day.

Use a red crayon to colour the number of hours that you are immobile, lying down or sitting. This includes sleeping, watching television (The minutes during which these activities are interrupted e.g. making a cup of tea, are not counted!), or films at the cinema, reading, using a computer, chatting to people, answering the telephone, driving a car or regular use of public transport.

Colour orange or yellow the hours that you spend on your feet. These include walking to the local shops or visiting a shopping mall, walking to visit family and friends, taking the stairs at work or going from one area to another, light housework and gardening, ironing, cooking, using the stairs at home. Add up the minutes and colour this time on the Mobility Pie diagram. These are your active hours.

The final colour is green. This represents exercise. Calculate the number of minutes and hours you devote to making your heart pump faster, getting out of breath, building your muscles. Exercise includes playing sports e.g. tennis, football, five-a-side, netball, hockey and golf, rock climbing, mountaineering and physical training; brisk walking, hiking, swimming, wrestling, working out in the gym, cycling on the road, or on an exercise bike, dancing and horse riding. Include chair exercises if you are injured or unable to walk.

If there is still blank space on your diagram, rethink your red area. Do you sleep longer or more often than you thought, watch television, read or write more often? Perhaps the yellow area needs to be expanded. Do you spend more time on your feet than you realise, but cannot remember exactly how much? Did you count the minutes immediately after getting up in the morning until sitting down for breakfast or in the car? You may have a mystery to solve. Just where does that lost time go?

When the diagram is completely coloured with no blank spaces, You will be able to to it in your notebook. You can use single words as well as sentences to catch thoughts and feelings about what has been revealed. Did you expect it to look differently, perhaps with more yellow areas? Are you shocked at how small the green area is? Perhaps you are pleased with a well-balanced circle.

By now you have a clear picture from your use of a pedometer and the record in your notebook, of how much walking you fit into your daily life. Walking, if you are able, is the most accessible and least costly form of exercise. It is very often the one activity that participants use as a starting point to increase their fitness. Walking is also the activity that is most likely to give the quickest results to people who do not do any other exercise or activity at all. These results may include the satisfYou will be able to of having seeing that you have made a start, enjoying being outside with a purpose, a sense of increasing physical fitness, sleeping better and appreciation of time to be away from responsibilities and time to think in peace.

Maintaining your incentive to walk is easier if you have a regular day, time and route to establish the habit. Having a destination has encouraged many participants. Visiting a friend lends an added purpose to the walk. Shopping malls are favourite destinations. Several hours of walking pose no problems when your attention is on the shops! Dogs are a great asset - if they are keen on exercise!

Spend some time remembering the activities you used to enjoy. Is it possible to take them up again? Are there facilities near to where you live or work, such as community centres, fitness clubs, dance classes? If you do not want to go alone, are there any friends, colleagues, relatives or neighbours that you could invite along?

Exercising with other people is often more enjoyable and the commitment to being part of a group can get you out of the house on the days you are reluctant to go out. But if all this seems too huge a leap, make your change smaller. Restrict yourself this week to making enquiries about what is available, which activities your friends take part in, the cost, times of opening, introductory offers. Simply using the week to familiarise yourself with exercise opportunities and imagining yourself taking part, in the same way as you prepared for this course, will make it easier to act the following week.

Making a small change at week 6

Choose a small change that will increase your level of movement or challenge you to raise your game to a higher level. Remember this has to fit into the context of your life and may require a reduction of, for example, red area immobility, such as watching television, in order to incorporate the new or increased activities. Don't forget to continue increasing your pedometer count.

Week 7 alcohol
Star Check

If you have chosen a small change in your portion sizes and completed that change once or more times last week, award yourself a star! If you have increased your steps, add another one. If you have made more than one change, take a bonus star!

You will be able to

- be able to calculate the number of units in alcoholic drinks
- understand the effects of alcohol
- understand levels of intoxication and sobering up times
- recognise the myths and truths about drinking

Week 7 Action

Drinking alcohol by choice in any form, may not be an intoxication issue for you. It may however be a factor in your weight gain, headaches or effect on long term health. To be in control and responsible for your personal health, it is helpful to have all the information relating to alcohol and its effects. This will ensure that you always have the foundation on which to make a choice.

We have provided material with which you can test your current knowledge. This always surprises most of our Small Changes course participants. It works both ways; amazing us about how much we don't know and how much we do. Try not to cheat by looking at the answers first. The time taken on Small Changes exercises and material is training time for your brain. It installs that necessary familiarity, in the same way as rehearsals for a play, a team game or a speech to be delivered. It positively effects your comprehension and recall and it is easier than rote learning.

Research into the difference between expert and amateur chess players, discovered that it was largely based on one factor. The experts played more often than the amateurs. Which seems to support the old adage that `practice makes perfect' or at least better.

Complete the truth/myth exercise and record your score in the notebook. This will enable you to compare your knowledge by repeating the exercise at some later date.

Read through Alcohol and the Brain, also The Binge Effect.

Using the size of wine glass that you normally use, pour out the amount you usually drink. Go to http://www.nhs.uk/Tools/Pages/Alcohol-unit-calculator.aspx where there is an Alcohol Unit Measurer tool. This will enable you to calculate unit sizes, compare them to the amount you assume you are pouring out. The tool can be downloaded to your computer for further use. The site also answers frequently asked questions about alcohol.

Drinking is a very personal issue and if you dislike alcohol these exercises and information may only be of cursory interest to you. Alternatively, if you have more complicated issues around alcohol that you feel you need help with, for yourself or your family, consider contacting the organisations that can guide you; on-line if you prefer to be anonymous, or by telephone is you want to discuss your own situation.

Making a Small Change at week 7

Choose a change that you feel will give you the highest benefit and remember not to be more ambitious that you are confident. If a change in alcohol consumption is a frightening challenge, make sure it is so small that you can achieve it instantly.

If you are satisfied with the amount and frequency of alcohol in your life, you can pass on this change! Remember to maintain or increase the changes you have already made.

Week 8 Relapse

Star Check

If you made a change, no matter how small, award yourself a star! If you have increased other changes, add another star. If you have made more than one change, take a bonus star!

You will be able to

- o   recognise the mechanics of relapse
- o   be aware of triggers
- o   be able to adopt and new position on the interpretation of relapses

Week 8 Action

Change is an unavoidable, constant part of human life. Everything we do – interacting socially, learning, getting ideas, maturing, growing older. What is this fear and avoidance of 'change'? Where does that blunt 'Can't change that mate..' attitude come from?

It is incomprehensible that we not only avoid change, but do not believe we are capable of it. There are moments in every period of change when we revert to the way we were. This is described as 'falling off the wagon', which indicates that we do have a language that embraces change, at least its failure. It feels like a shameful incompetency that prompts all those self-doubts to clamber back into our minds. Are we lacking in backbone and tenacity? Are we weak characters with no real determination? Does this 'always happen to me'?

Yes it does. It happens to everyone. It happens to people who are deliberately changing their way of life, perhaps from smoking, over eating or losing their temper. If they fail and return to smoking, over-eating and initiating a ruckus, they call it 'relapse'.

In Small Changes we do not believe in relapse in terms of ceasing to change. There are moments in every period of change when we revert to the way we were. The fact is, change is happening most of the time and reverting back to the way life used to live is totally normal behaviour. It is *part* of changing, not the opposite of changing.

We asked one group of eight Small Changes group participants how many years they had been attending weight control sessions. The answer was 142. These women were expert weight losers. . They had of course been repeatedly successful in achieving their main goal of losing weight and just as successful in putting it back on, plus some.

Losing weight and changing your lifestyle are two different goals. The first may be short term and temporary, the second is on-going and permanent.

Revisiting the way we were, is not a simple need to 'get back to normal' after stringent dieting. It is not about needing to be back the easy, safe and unchallenging place. People that have worked at changing, feel good about the results. They want it to continue. In fact they expect it to continue as the new 'normal'.

However, everyone can be caught unawares by a trigger. Revisiting the way we were can be caused when one thing reminds you of another and precipitates an old memory you will be able to remember an old association.

- Tea = biscuits   Nobody dunks biscuits in a cup of water
- Meal in a restaurant = at least three courses regardless of other meals that day
- Driving home = chocolate from the petrol station
- Watching TV = crisps and sweets
- Seaside = ice-cream

Keep an eye on yourself this week and notice the number of times that you are attracted to food or drink that you used to like, but have stopped buying because you are now making healthier choices e.g. more often fruit salad than sticky toffee pudding. Make a note of old habits calling to you and try to identify the trigger that has roused the old habits.

If you succumb, it is not the crime of the century. Nor is it a relapse. Neither does make you a failure. It is a return to the way you were, triggered off by a physical or emotional association. To become immune to these triggers you need to practice recognising them and develop ways to avoid reacting.

Making a small change at week 8

Read through your record of triggers that send you back to the way you were. They can have occurred this week, or be others that you are wary of. Devise on one avoidance method and practice that way of avoiding the pull to return to the way you were. You could practice by deliberately going to places where you know there will be a trigger. Make a note of your strategy.

Week 9   Review and evaluate

Star Check

If you created a strategy to counteract a trigger, you have earned a gold star. If it worked, take a second gold star!

You will be able to appreciate how much effort and energy you have used to achieve your success

- o see how much your confidence and commitment to your health has increased
- o know how to maintain your new normal
- o feel responsible and able to be in control of your of your health
- o plan how to celebrate your successes

Week 9 Action

It is now time to revisit your mountain and mark the place to which you have climbed.

On your rating page, circle the number you feel you have achieved in confidence and motivation. Look through your notebook and remember the weeks in which you made changes. Count those stars........

Future Strategies and Celebration

You will be able to

- o plan how to celebrate your successes
- o look forward to making changes in any area of your life
- o use the Small Changes techniques to increase changes if you need to
- o be able to select techniques if you need to re-focus and maintain weight loss
- o realise that you have proved that you are a responsible person who is knowledgeable about and in control of their own health

Making a small change at week 9

It is resolution time... if you had to make just one resolution for the future, what would it be? Write it in your notebook and during the next few weeks' notice how many times you act on that resolution.

Star Check

Two stars for making a resolution and acting on it and five more for completing the Solo Small Changes course! Congratulations! You deserve a standing ovation and a bouquet for that performance!

The future

The new normal that you have reached can be elaborated by additional changes that suit your lifestyle. Keep some gold stars to award yourself! If you lose some momentum, look back over the course material and re-introduce the techniques that worked well for you and you feel will get you back on track.

If you start to worry about eating regularly, complete a food diary for a week and assess the size of the problem. It may not be as bad as you think and you can change it just as you did before.

You can continue to make changes e.g. reducing or increasing food, adding to or trying new physical activities or increasing your support by encouraging more friends to join you.

The present

Regarded as the most influential scientist in history, Isaac Newton, who discovered the laws of gravity, commented on his achievements 'If I have seen further, it is only by standing on the shoulders of giants.'

His `giants' were the scientists who had gone before, those who showed the way.

Our giants are also those who have gone before. They are the people who have lost weight and continue to maintain that loss. We know how, and are successful at losing weight, but not very successful at keeping it off.

We *do* know what most people who have lost weight and maintain that loss do. Our giants are 'ordinary' folk who took control of their health, as you have done over the past nine weeks. The method has been discovered by asking individual people how they succeeded and keeping track of them for years.

Although the range of differences between people is wide, there are common denominators that apply to them all – the 'most people' principle. Naturally the range of achievement is also wide as it partly depends on the individual starting point and on personal goals.

The National Weight Control Registry of America has a membership of which 80% of persons are women and 20% are men. The members have lost an average of 66 lbs

(4st 10lb) and kept it off for five and a half years up to now.

These are averages, within which there is a lot of diversity. Weight losses have ranged from 30lbs (2st 2lb) to 300 lbs (21st 6lb). The duration of maintaining this weight loss has ranged from 1 year to 66 years.

The NWCR has also started to learn about how the weight loss was accomplished.

- 45% of registry participants lost the weight on their own
- 55% lost weight with the help of some type of programme
- some people have lost the weight rapidly
- others have lost weight very slowly over as many as 14 years

And here is the crux – most people succeed by changing their food intake and level of physical activity.

- 98% of registry participants modified their food intake in some way
- 94% increased their physical activity, with the most frequently reported form of activity being walking

How do most people do this?

- ✓ 78% eat breakfast every day
- ✓ 75% weigh themselves at least once a week to keep a check on progress
- ✓ 62% watch less than 10 hours of TV per week
- ✓ 90% exercise, on average, for about 1 hour per day

Most members maintain a low calorie, low fat diet and do higher levels of activity than they did prior to losing weight. Small Changes participants only make changes that fit into the context of their current lifestyle. Every change is chosen by the individual according to what they feel is the most important issue for them. Our approach totally personal and is designed to include every aspect of a participant's life, because every part of our lives interrelates and effects the whole. In short, real life is not consistently regular or organised. Unexpected events occur, accidents happen, schedules change and routines are disrupted.

By choosing the Small Changes that are feasible for them, the individual remains in control of their health decisions and will experience continuous success. A disruption of routine is just that, something to deal with, to negotiate around, to accept until it passes.

APPENDIX ONE

Chapter 1 Assessment Answers

1=F, 2=T, 3=T, 4=T, 5=F, 6=T, 7=T, 8=F. 9=F

Chapter 2 Assessment Answers

1. At the core of a comprehensive programme: food, physical activity *and* behaviour all should be covered

2. A programme might usefully run forever and weight-management is a chronic lifelong condition... but your funder might have different views! Running a programme ad infinitum will be difficult to justify from a cost-effectiveness point of view. Perhaps we will discover in time that around a year is optimum? There may be no extra benefit from extending to two years- see Perri references around length of treatment

3. Participants come to us all the time with stories about how they spent the week exercising and eating well only to discover they had not changed or even gained weight! Please convince them to only weigh without clothes/minimal clothes, first thing in the morning after going to the toilet and before eating or drinking anything. This will give an accurate picture of their weight that will fluctuate greatly through the day- other measure like waist circumference and a body-compositional analyser will give a 'triangulation' of results that is better than weight alone.

4. Increased fruit and veg consumption, increased fitness or number of minutes of physical activity are all worth celebrating/ independent ameliorators of disease risk- irrespective of weight loss- let's broaden our horizons and those of the participants to encompass all positive changes and not just bodyweight alone.

Key criticism from a public health perspective would be the likelihood that these changes would be reversed after the intervention has finished- difficult though it is we need to work towards sustained change, We can start to talk about 'long-term' change when results are shown at one-year and post-one year.

Chapter 3 Assessment Answers

1=F, 2=T , 3= T, 4 = F

Chapter 4 Assessment Answers

1=T, 2= T, 3=T,4=T,5=F,

Chapter 5 Assessment Answers

1. True. Increased intake of calorie-dense foods may provide some people with extra glucose needed by the brain in times of stress. Obesity may result when the brain is unable to demand and receive glucose from the body efficiently.

2. True. Our distant ancestors ate ripe fruits with a high fructose content in the autumn to provide an immediate energy source and increase fat stores for the winter.

3. Higher intakes of fat and total calories and higher BMI.

4. It is a myth that you need special products to detoxify your body. Your liver, kidneys, intestines, lungs and skin get rid of waste matter and toxins very efficiently every day helped by regular exercise and a balanced, healthy diet.

5. False. Unlike most modern Western diets it was alkaline and potassium-rich with twice as much fruit and vegetable intake.

6. True. Good bone strength and density depends on having adequate muscle mass, which means eating enough high-quality protein. Higher protein diets are associated with greater bone mass and fewer fractures, provided calcium intake is adequate.

Chapter 6 Assessment Answers

1. False/Nonsense! if a person who walks two minutes a day does four it's a hundred percent increase... the client needs to take control over what they do with your facilitation- they will decide what is too much or enough

2. True/ In a paper by Schneider et al. in 2006 there is a good example of how the 'behaviour' of walking 10,000 steps a day can affect people's weight and other indices of health positively

3. True- this is the point the 60 mins a day/10,000 steps guidelines are really useful when a client asks for them (and they do *sometimes* ask for them) but it is really what the client feels/how much they feel is feasible to do that is important and this stems from self-awareness around their current physical activity.

Chapter 7 Assessment Answers

1=T, 2=T

Chapter 8 Assessment Answers

1. Simple and Complex
2. Complex
3. F
4. T
5. T
6. Empathy

APPENDIX 2

TOOLS FOR SUCCESSFUL BEHAVIOUR CHANGE

As self-awareness or raising the client's awareness is a key goal in behaviour change (so that they are in a better position to make decisions) tools for successful behaviour change reflect this. These are ways of looking at what a client does (or what you do yourself) and giving time to reflect on this.

1. A Day in the Life

'A day in the life' is a good example; here the client is invited to tell you what happens from when they get out of bed and to when they get back into it. How they eat, what they do with their time what activities fill their day. There will be insight into what kind if lifestyle they have as a result and naturally the person needs to recall what happens and how their time is spent. A piece of paper used as a day in the life diary can help but this can also be done verbally. Follow-on open questions and elaborations will help fill in the picture.

'You say you do… what is that like?'

Equally using summaries and reflections will be useful to show you are listening and to ensure your own attention. 1-10 scales as used in MI are a useful way of assessing importance. On a scale on 1-10 how important is this issue to you? and then as a follow on:

'You say four; I wonder why this is not as important as say 6 or 7'

2. Activity wheel

Using the activity wheel, introduced in the physical activity chapter (page 126) is a useful way of people looking at how they spend the time, lack of time is a very common explanation for why people cannot be physically active. If that I so it is a great idea to look as 24 hours in a person's typical day to see what happens to all that time. Very often in Small Changes people discover a lot of red or orange time (time that is spent completely sedentary or only doing very energy-inexpensive activity such as sitting at a desk or driving).

3. Pedometers

Pedometers are excellent awareness raising tools- even if they are not calibrated to very sensitively pick up exact step numbers (an issues many of our clients find frustrating) they do pick up *relative* changes. So instead of exact number of steps you end of with an obvious sign of increasing steps- if the pedometer under-counts it will still do so when steps increase but the increase will be evident.

4. Wheel of life

The wheel of life is about assessing where people are in relation to their whole life and can help identify the client's priorities. Sections can include work-satisfaction, love-life, diet, exercise, friendships, finance and relationships etc. The wheel of Life is commonly used in Neuro Linguistic Programming and is a tool we've encountered at various training courses. The idea is that people evaluate their life 'balance' and identify areas of greatest satisfaction/concern.

The wheel is not a scientific tool but rather a useful awareness raising device to help people look at where the imbalance is in their life and to explore how important this is and discover what they want to do about it.

5. Label reading cards

We have developed our own Small Changes label reading card (there are many) you can have free access to the one provided here. The key elements are looking at the per 100grams section of a label. This really makes sense if you figure something that contains 5 grams of fat per 100 grams of product is 5% fat.

The essential idea here is not to interpret the card as saying you should never eat products that don't meet the guidelines for healthy (god forbid or I'd never be able to eat cheesecake again!) the idea moreover is to fill your weeks shopping basket and look at where most products fit. Vegetables are givens in that they always fit even the few exceptions that are higher are higher in essential fatty acids and unsaturated fatty acids. So bung them in (and there are no labels anyway but for this exercise we'll assume they all meet the 'good' criteria). After this you'll find massive variance and the card can help you when there is an array of products to pick the one you think is best.

Low-fat varieties could be a complicated area- I personally make the choice to eat the full-fat variety of many food s that are treat foods but eat them very sparingly. Others, however, might want to eat these foods more often and try the lower-fat varieties to reduce their Kcalorie intake. I feel the nutritionist ion me taking over and will move on…

6. Support

Support seems to be the ultimate issue with Small Changes. People are not overweight because they do not know that eating high Kcalorie food and being inactive cause an energy imbalance. There may be information they do want about exercise and nutrition and self-awareness is often a stumbling block to realising what's going on. Success, however, on our programmes seems to come from the support clients feel they are getting in making their own lifestyle choices which ultimately help them become more physically active and eat better. Sustaining this support seems crucial if we are to maintain lifestyle changes for the long-term.

Attending a class each week where people will listen empathically and be interested is inherently supportive in research giving people attention and support in this way might be described as the Hawthorn effect. In behaviour change the Hawthorne effect is a good thing! Not merely a way of suggesting your intervention is not what has made the effect but rather a placebo type effect that is not actually the food, the drug the exercise or whatever it is that you are testing. If you could bottle this type of attention you'd be on to a winner.

Client would do well to obtain a good support system! Who will listen to them? Is there anyone in their life that is a good empathic listener? The responsibility for moving forward and changing remains with the person who wants to change but good support is essential.

These sentence stems might be a good starting point for letting someone know how good their support is:

Thinking if the support you would like to receive how might you complete these sentences to a friend or loved one who may potentially support you with weight-management?

> *I like it when you…*
>
> *I find it supportive when…*
>
> *You may not realise this but It really helps me when you just…*

Here the client is offered the chance to affirm or support the person giving support- a virtuous circle!

> *I like it when you just listen to me.*

Anatomy of a small change

Participants on a Small Changes course want to lose weight. This is not a throw-away generalisation, but a conclusion we have reached over a number of years.

Although a variety of reasons are offered by participants – from wanting to make the 'right' food choices, to feeling less tired and able play with their toddlers – the unequivocal aim is to lose weight.

This is their primary aim and none of the side-effects such as gaining a waist or feeling younger and in control of their health, come anywhere near the importance of losing weight. Even maintenance of weight loss is often not part of the initial conversation about what they expect from Small Changes.

Small Changes course facilitators aim to manage participants' expectations by enabling them to experience losing weight.

Recognition

Making a series of small lifestyle changes that will result in permanent alterations in choice, taste, experience, needs and self-management, starts with the recognition of every participant as a unique individual. Each person has their own history of life experiences, which influences their desires and decisions.

They come to the group with very personal agendas. Imagine these stuffed into a handbag, plonked on the table and opened at random. Stories are told, memories shared, people are laughing, expressing surprise and sympathy. Contents of the handbags are easily spilled out and enjoyed, because they are recognisable as common and enjoyable to share; light anecdotes that have been in and out of the handbags many times.

Under the table, each participant has placed a suitcase containing the real weight of their experience that is not comical or presentable to strangers. Within the suitcase are the reasons that dictate their owners' life choices. Some of the contents have been forgotten, or are not recognised by the suitcase owner as influential. Much of the pain, grief and guilt lies underneath these contents, making choice and change extremely difficult and complicated.

Method

A successful method of change has four qualities.

- Choice of action made exclusively by participant
- Small (number of times, duration, quantity) size change
- Fitting within the context of participant's life
- Anchored to specific date, time, number, duration, company

Example:

Wendy wants to increase the steps recorded on her pedometer. She has been shocked by the average of 1,000 steps per day recorded during her first week with a pedometer. She suggests walking every day until 2,000 steps have been recorded.

NB   This is a 100% increase in activity for this woman.
She aims to do it every day.
If Wendy misses a day or more, she will feel a failure.

Questions:

Where does she intend to walk? To a destination e.g. sister's house?

- Who with?

- Exactly what time will she walk? How long will it take?
- Will she want to walk if the weather is cold or it is raining?
- Are there places to walk that Wendy feels are safe?
- What activity will she have to drop in order to make time to walk?
- Does she have comfortable shoes to walk in?
- Will Wendy find walking boring or are there interesting views/plants?
- What else would put her off going out every day?
- Is there anyone who will encourage her to keep it up?
-

Having explored all the answers it will become possible to fit Wendy's chosen small change into the context of her life.

Conclusion:

100% increase in anything is likely to be too much to sustain, especially if the participant does not already go out walking just for exercise. Two walks can be agreed and regarded as a successful increase in steps. If more walks are taken they can be applauded as 'extra' success.

It is likely that she does not enjoy walking for the sake of walking, but having a destination e.g. sister's house, gives purpose and enjoyment in their meeting.

When exactly will Wendy walk to her sister's house? Tuesday and Thursday afternoons at 2-4pm her sister is at home with the baby and Wendy usually speaks to her on the telephone. Wendy can do her gardening in the mornings instead of those afternoons.

She has past experience of her sister's neighbourhood and knows the route to her house very well. She enjoys being in the neighbourhood where she used to live and feels safe there. Her husband will probably tease her about walking, but he is already very encouraging about her effort to be healthier.

Proposed small change:

Wendy will do two walks, alone, to her sister's house at 2pm on Tuesday and Thursday.

Rationale:

Two is a small, achievable number that fit into the context of Wendy's current timetable. It allows for inclement weather conditions and gives time to change days or time within the week. Walking with a destination is easier than a route. Wendy enjoys talking to her sister and her husband is already supportive.

Check: for method of change qualities

- Choice of action made exclusively by participant
- Small (number of times, duration, quantity) size change
- Fitting within the context of participant's life
- Anchored to specific date, time, number, duration, company

Conclusion:

Wendy will leave the session knowing exactly what, when and where she is going to make a realistic small change. There are no other decisions to make and no doubt or question about whether she will make the change. She will avoid the '*I can do it tomorrow*' and 'There is plenty of time at the end of the week' or 'I don't feel like walking today' dilemmas...

At the next group session she will enjoy sharing her success and relating her feelings of achievement and confidence in herself.

INDEX